Nomad

**Silent Currents: Navigating the Hidden Dangers of
Electromagnetic Fields (EMF)**

Nomad

Silent Currents: Navigating the Hidden Dangers of
Electromagnetic Fields (EMF)

Copyright © *Levitas One*, 2024

All Rights Reserved

What are the NoMAD Plans?

Developed by Dr Ash Kapoor, the NoMAD Plans represent a transformative approach to health and wellness that combines the wisdom of ancestral practices with contemporary medical insights. The name "NoMAD" not only suggests a journey through the intricate realm of health but also stands for its foundational principles: Nutritional Optimisation, Mindful Adaptation, and Detoxification.

At the heart of NoMAD is the 6R Framework—Restore, Release, Repair, Renew, Reframe, and Represent. This methodology addresses the root causes of illness, combats chronic inflammation, and cultivates authentic vitality, guiding individuals through a transformative process.

Tailored specifically to each individual, NoMAD journeys are meticulously crafted to rebalance the body, strengthen the mind, and rejuvenate overall health. By integrating ancestral practices with cutting-edge, innovative treatments—all under strict medical oversight—NoMAD Plans offer a personalised pathway to sustainable, long-lasting health and wellness that resonates with your unique life circumstances.

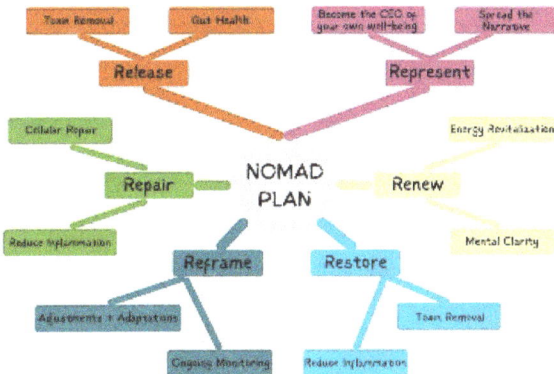

Levitas One:
"As Is In, As Is Out"

Reflecting the belief that our internal health and wellness is mirrored in our external environment. Founded by Dr. Ash Kapoor, Levitas One serves as the vehicle for delivering NoMAD's treatment plans. It envisions a healthcare future where patients are at the centre of a fully integrated, multidisciplinary approach. Guided by Nomads 6 Rs—Restore, Release, Repair, Renew, Reframe, and Represent—Levitas One empowers self-care through personalised guidance and minimal intervention, promoting long-term health, balance, and sustainability.

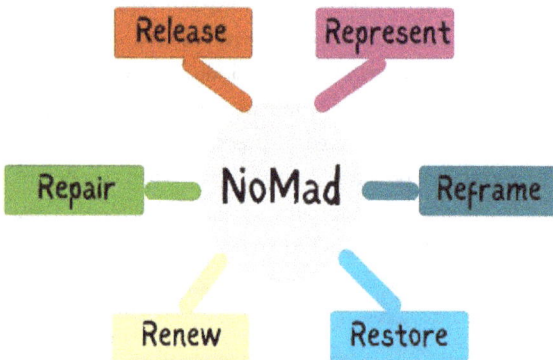

Release   Represent

Repair ← NoMad → Reframe

Renew   Restore

Contents

Preface

In my 35-year career in medicine, I have witnessed a profound transformation in how we live, work, and interact within society. The advent of information automation has ushered in an era characterised by unprecedented speed and convenience, redefining the boundaries of our daily lives. Information is now delivered at lightning speed, channeled through multiple sources simultaneously, and seamlessly integrated into our routines. While this digital evolution has brought numerous advantages, it has also introduced a hidden layer of toxicity and complex challenges that were once inconceivable.

Our modern environments, saturated with electromagnetic fields (EMF) from countless electronic devices, wireless networks, and smart technologies, are creating an invisible threat to human health and health and wellness. This pervasive exposure, combined with the demands of constant connectivity, has led to what I term "the new era of toxicity." It is an era that brings with it unique stressors, affecting not only our physical health but also our psychological resilience and quality of life.

This book aims to address these invisible threats and provide actionable solutions. It draws from the latest scientific research, insights from the Human Optimisation Conference, and my personal experiences over the past decade, attending various courses and exploring different approaches to health and wellness. By combining evidence-based strategies with a holistic view of health and wellness, I hope to offer a comprehensive guide that empowers readers to reclaim their health in a technology-driven world.

Through this book, I seek to illuminate the less obvious impacts of modern living and provide practical advice on how to navigate this complex landscape. I believe that by acknowledging and addressing these challenges, we can move towards a healthier, more balanced life in harmony with our rapidly changing environment.

Chapter 1
Electromagnetic Fields (EMF) and Health Impact

Overview of EMF: Definition and Classification

Electromagnetic fields (EMF) are invisible areas of energy, often referred to as radiation, that are associated with the use of electrical power and various forms of naturally and man-made lighting. EMFs are produced by the movement of electrically charged particles and are present all around us, both in natural and human-made environments. The Earth's natural electromagnetic field is generated by the movement of molten metal within its core, while human-made EMFs are produced by electrical appliances, power lines, wireless networks, and communication devices like cell phones and laptops.

The term EMF encompasses a broad spectrum of electromagnetic radiation, ranging from extremely low frequencies (ELF) produced by power lines and electrical appliances to higher-frequency fields like those produced by microwaves, X-rays, and gamma rays. The energy carried by an EMF depends on its frequency and wavelength. Higher frequency EMFs have shorter wavelengths and carry more energy, while lower frequency EMFs have longer wavelengths and carry less energy. Understanding the different types and sources of EMF is crucial for assessing their potential health impacts.

Health concerns regarding EMF exposure have emerged with the increasing use of electronic devices and the proliferation of wireless technologies. Researchers are investigating whether prolonged exposure to low-level EMFs can cause adverse health effects, particularly for vulnerable populations such as children and pregnant women. Understanding the basic science of EMF is the first step in evaluating its impact on health and implementing strategies to mitigate potential risks.

Types of EMF: Ionising vs. Non-Ionising

The electromagnetic spectrum is divided into two primary categories: **ionising radiation** and **non-ionising radiation**. These two types of EMF differ significantly in their energy levels and potential to cause harm.

1. Ionising Radiation:

Ionising radiation has enough energy to remove tightly bound electrons from atoms, a process known as ionisation. This type of radiation can cause direct damage to DNA and cellular structures, leading to potential health issues such as cancer. Ionising radiation includes:

- **X-rays**: Commonly used in medical imaging, X-rays have high energy and can penetrate the human body to create detailed images of internal organs and bones. While beneficial for diagnostic purposes, repeated exposure to high levels of X-rays can increase the risk of cancer.
- **Gamma rays**: Gamma rays are emitted from radioactive materials and certain cosmic sources. They are highly penetrating and can cause significant damage to living tissue, making them a concern in radiation therapy and nuclear safety.
- **Ultraviolet (UV) radiation**: UV radiation, which comes from sunlight, is on the border between ionising and non-ionising radiation. It has enough energy to damage skin cells and DNA, leading to skin ageing and an increased risk of skin cancer.

2. Non-Ionising Radiation:

Non-ionising radiation has lower energy and longer wavelengths compared to ionising radiation. It does not have enough energy to remove electrons from atoms or directly damage DNA. Non-ionising radiation includes:

- **Extremely Low Frequency (ELF) Radiation**: Produced by power lines, electrical wiring, and appliances like refrigerators and washing machines. ELF radiation has very low energy and is not considered a major health risk at typical exposure levels.
- **Radiofrequency (RF) Radiation**: Emitted by wireless devices like cell phones, Wi-Fi routers, and Bluetooth devices. RF radiation has higher energy than ELF but is still considered low compared to ionising radiation.
- **Microwave Radiation**: Used in microwave ovens and certain communication devices. While it can heat water molecules, it does not ionise atoms or molecules in the body.
- **Visible Light**: The light we see is a form of non-ionising radiation. It is essential for vision but has little impact on health at typical exposure levels.

Understanding the distinction between ionising and non-ionising radiation helps clarify which types of EMF pose a greater risk to health. While non-ionising radiation is generally considered safer, concerns about chronic exposure to lower energy fields, such as those from cell phones and Wi-Fi routers, have prompted further research.

Common Sources of EMF Exposure

Electromagnetic fields (EMF) are present in our environment from both natural and artificial sources. While the Earth's magnetic field is a natural source of low-level EMF, human-made sources contribute significantly to our daily EMF exposure. Understanding these common sources can help us identify potential risks and implement strategies to reduce exposure.

Natural Sources of EMF:

- **Earth's Magnetic Field**: The Earth generates a constant magnetic field that protects us from solar radiation. This natural EMF is part of our environment and has no known harmful effects at typical levels.
- **Cosmic and Solar Radiation**: Space emits low levels of ionising radiation in the form of gamma rays and cosmic rays. The atmosphere shields us from most of these harmful rays, but exposure increases at high altitudes and during air travel.

Human-Made Sources of EMF:

- **Power Lines and Electrical Wiring**: Power lines and the electrical wiring in homes and offices produce extremely low-frequency (ELF) EMFs. These fields are strongest close to the source and diminish with distance.
- **Electronic Devices and Appliances**: Everyday appliances such as refrigerators, hair dryers, microwaves, and washing machines emit ELF and RF radiation. EMF exposure from these devices is usually low and limited to times when they are in use.
- **Wireless Communication Devices**: Mobile phones, Wi-Fi routers, and Bluetooth devices emit radiofrequency (RF) radiation. The widespread use of these devices has increased concern about long-term health effects, especially when devices are kept close to the body, such as carrying a phone in a pocket or using wireless earbuds.
- **Medical Equipment**: MRI machines and other medical devices that use high-frequency radiation can expose patients and healthcare workers to higher levels of EMF.

With the proliferation of wireless technologies and electronic devices, our exposure to EMF has increased exponentially. This makes it essential to understand the sources and levels of exposure to make informed decisions about reducing potential risks.

Summary: Electromagnetic Fields (EMF) and Health Impact

(a) EMF Overview

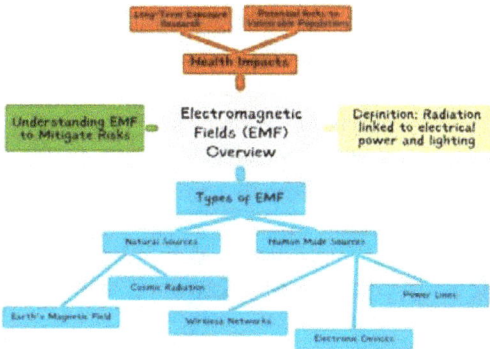

(b) Types of EMF

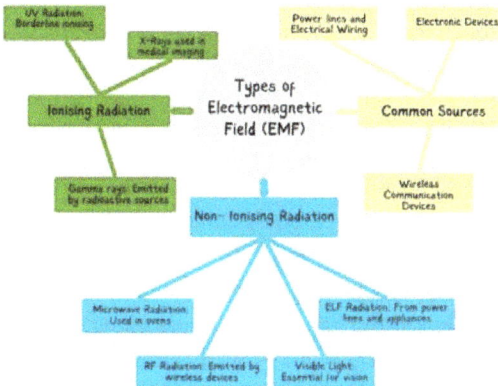

Chapter 2
Health Effects of EMF Exposure

The health effects of EMF exposure are a topic of ongoing research and debate. While high-frequency ionising radiation is known to cause harm, such as DNA damage and cancer, the potential health impacts of low-frequency non-ionising radiation are less clear. Some studies suggest that chronic exposure to low levels of EMF may contribute to a variety of health issues, while others find no significant risks.

Biological Mechanisms: How EMF Affects the Body

Research indicates that non-ionising EMFs, such as those from cell phones and Wi-Fi, interact with biological tissues in several ways. One proposed mechanism is the generation of oxidative stress, where free radicals are produced, leading to cellular damage and inflammation. Another mechanism involves calcium channel activation, which may disrupt cellular signalling. However, these interactions are still not fully understood and require more investigation.

Short-term vs. Long-term Exposure

Short-term exposure to EMF is generally considered safe at typical environmental levels. For instance, using a microwave or cell phone for a few minutes poses little risk. However, long-term exposure, especially at higher levels, is of greater concern. Studies on long-term exposure, such as residential proximity to power lines, have shown mixed results, with some suggesting an increased risk of childhood leukemia and others showing no significant association.

Health Risks of Ionising Radiation

Ionising radiation, such as that from X-rays and gamma rays, is a known carcinogen. It has enough energy to break chemical bonds, leading to DNA damage and potentially cancer. Exposure to ionising radiation is carefully regulated, especially in medical settings, to minimise health risks.

Health Risks of Non-Ionising Radiation

The potential health risks of non-ionising radiation are less clear. Some epidemiological studies have suggested associations between long-term RF exposure and an increased risk of brain tumours, but these findings are inconsistent. Concerns have also been raised about reproductive health, neurological effects, and changes in sleep patterns. However, the evidence is not strong enough to establish causation.

Vulnerable Populations: Children and Pregnant Women

Children and pregnant women may be more susceptible to EMF exposure due to their developing systems. Children's thinner skulls and greater tissue conductivity mean they absorb more RF energy from devices like cell phones. Similarly, prenatal exposure to EMF could potentially affect fetal development. Precautionary measures, such as limiting children's use of wireless devices, are recommended until more conclusive research is available.

Clinical Case Study: 35-year-old IT Professional with Chronic Headaches and Fatigue

A 35-year-old male, working as an IT professional, reported experiencing chronic headaches, fatigue, and difficulty concentrating over the past year. His job required him to spend 8–10 hours daily surrounded by multiple screens, Wi-Fi routers, and other electronic devices. The patient noticed his symptoms worsened during the workweek and improved on weekends when he was less exposed to electronic devices.

A thorough medical evaluation ruled out underlying conditions like migraines or vision problems. Suspecting a link to chronic EMF exposure, the healthcare provider recommended practical changes: taking regular breaks from screens, increasing distance from Wi-Fi routers, and turning off non-essential devices. Additionally, the patient was advised to turn off his home Wi-Fi router at night and limit his use of wireless devices after work.

After three months of implementing these changes, the patient reported a significant reduction in the frequency and severity of his headaches and improved overall energy levels. Although it's difficult to attribute these improvements solely to reduced EMF exposure, the case suggests that lifestyle adjustments can positively impact health and health and wellness in individuals experiencing similar symptoms.

Health Effects of EMF Exposure

Biological Mechanisms: How EMF Affects the Body

Electromagnetic fields (EMF) interact with biological systems in several complex ways, depending on their frequency and energy level. The biological effects of EMF exposure can be categorised into thermal and non-thermal effects. **Thermal effects** occur when the energy from an EMF source is sufficient to increase the temperature of biological tissues. This is most commonly seen with high-frequency EMFs like microwaves, which can heat water molecules in the body, leading to localised tissue heating. While microwave ovens are designed to contain this energy, certain industrial or medical applications of high-frequency EMFs can pose risks if not properly controlled.

Non-thermal effects, which occur at lower energy levels (e.g., those from mobile phones, Wi-Fi, or power lines), are less understood and are the focus of ongoing research. These effects do not cause a temperature rise but may interfere with biological processes in more subtle ways. One proposed mechanism is the alteration of cellular ion channels, particularly calcium channels.

When exposed to EMF, these channels may allow excess calcium ions to enter cells, disrupting normal cellular function and potentially leading to oxidative stress.

Another proposed mechanism is the production of reactive oxygen species **(ROS)**, commonly known as free radicals. ROS are highly reactive molecules that can cause damage to proteins, lipids, and DNA within cells. Elevated levels of ROS have been linked to various health conditions, including inflammation, ageing, and cancer. Research suggests that chronic exposure to low-level EMFs may increase ROS production, leading to oxidative stress and subsequent cellular damage. However, the evidence for these effects is not yet conclusive, and more research is needed to understand the long-term implications fully.

Neurobiological effects of EMF exposure are also an area of active investigation. Some studies suggest that EMF exposure may alter neurotransmitter release or disrupt the blood-brain barrier, which protects the brain from harmful substances. These changes could theoretically contribute to symptoms such as headaches, dizziness, and cognitive difficulties reported by some individuals with high EMF exposure. However, these findings remain controversial and are not widely accepted by the scientific community.

Lastly, EMF exposure has been shown to influence **gene expression** in certain experimental models. Some studies indicate that low-level EMF exposure can alter the expression of genes involved in stress responses, apoptosis (programmed cell death), and DNA repair. These findings suggest that EMF exposure could potentially impact cellular health and function at a molecular level. Yet, translating these results into clinically relevant health outcomes remains challenging due to variability in study designs and exposure conditions.

In summary, while several biological mechanisms have been proposed to explain how EMF exposure affects the body, none are definitively proven in humans. The impact of EMF on health likely depends on the intensity, duration, and frequency of exposure, as well as individual susceptibility factors such as age, genetics, and pre-existing health conditions.

Acute vs. Chronic Exposure

The health effects of EMF exposure can differ significantly depending on whether the exposure is acute (short-term) or chronic (long-term). Understanding this distinction is essential for evaluating potential risks.

Acute exposure refers to short-term exposure to EMF at high levels. This can occur, for example, during medical imaging procedures like X-rays or MRI scans, or from sudden exposure to a high-powered electrical source. The primary concern with acute exposure is the potential for tissue heating and thermal damage. For instance, being exposed to high-frequency microwave radiation for a short period can cause localised heating of tissues, leading to burns or heat-induced damage. Regulatory agencies have established safety limits to prevent these acute thermal effects in occupational and medical settings.

Chronic exposure, on the other hand, involves lower levels of EMF over extended periods. This is the type of exposure most people experience from everyday sources like power lines, household appliances, and wireless devices. The potential health effects of chronic exposure are less well understood, primarily because non-ionising radiation from these sources does not have enough energy to cause direct DNA damage. However, some studies suggest that prolonged exposure to low-level EMF may contribute to long-term health issues such as sleep disturbances, cognitive changes, and increased risk of certain cancers. For example, epidemiological studies have linked long-term exposure to residential power lines with a slightly increased risk of childhood leukemia, though the evidence is not conclusive.

The difference between acute and chronic exposure also lies in how the body responds to EMF. Acute exposure may cause immediate symptoms such as headaches or disziness, whereas chronic exposure's effects may be delayed and more subtle. Chronic exposure's potential cumulative effect raises concerns about long-term health risks, especially for individuals who are exposed to higher levels of EMF at work or through heavy use of electronic devices.

Ultimately, while acute exposure risks are well understood and managed through safety standards, the risks associated with chronic, low-level exposure are still a matter of scientific debate and ongoing research.

Health Risks of Ionising Radiation

Ionising radiation is a form of electromagnetic radiation with enough energy to ionise atoms or molecules, which means it can remove tightly bound electrons, leading to chemical changes in cells. This type of radiation includes X-rays, gamma rays, and ultraviolet (UV) radiation. Due to its high energy, ionising radiation poses a significant risk to human health, particularly through its potential to cause DNA damage.

When DNA is damaged by ionising radiation, it can lead to mutations that may interfere with normal cell function. If the damage is not properly repaired, it can initiate carcinogenesis, the process by which normal cells become cancerous. This is why ionising radiation is classified as a **Group 1 carcinogen** by the International Agency for Research on Cancer (IARC). Frequent or high-level exposure to ionising radiation has been linked to an increased risk of various cancers, including leukemia, thyroid cancer, and breast cancer.

In medical settings, ionising radiation is used for diagnostic imaging and cancer treatment. While these applications are beneficial, they must be carefully managed to minimise the risk of harmful side effects. For example, X-rays are used to produce images of bones and organs, but repeated exposure can increase cancer risk. As a result, healthcare providers use the **"as low as** reasonably achievable" **(ALARA)** principle to limit radiation doses and protect both patients and medical staff.

Because of its potential to cause harm, ionising radiation exposure is regulated by safety standards that set maximum permissible levels for occupational and environmental exposure.

Health Risks of Non-Ionising Radiation

Non-ionising radiation, which includes extremely low-frequency (ELF) radiation, radiofrequency (RF) radiation, and microwaves, does not carry enough energy to ionise atoms or molecules. This lower energy level makes non-ionising radiation generally less hazardous than ionising radiation. However, concerns remain about its potential health effects, especially with long-term exposure to sources like mobile phones, Wi-Fi routers, and power lines.

The most widely discussed potential health risks associated with non-ionising radiation are related to **radiofrequency (RF) radiation**, which is emitted by wireless devices like cell phones, tablets, and Wi-Fi routers. Some studies have suggested that prolonged exposure to RF radiation, particularly when mobile phones are used close to the head, may increase the risk of developing brain tumours such as gliomas or acoustic neuromas. However, these studies have limitations, including recall bias and small sample sizes, and the overall evidence is inconsistent. The World Health Organisation (WHO) has classified RF radiation as a **"possible human carcinogen" (Group 2B)**, indicating that while there is some evidence of risk, it is not conclusive.

Non-ionising radiation has also been implicated in other health effects, such as sleep disturbances, headaches, and reduced sperm quality. For example, studies have shown that individuals who use their mobile phones for extended periods may experience more frequent headaches and report poorer sleep quality. Similarly, exposure to RF radiation has been associated with decreased sperm motility and viability in some animal studies.

Overall, while non-ionising radiation is considered less harmful than ionising radiation, concerns about its potential health effects have led to precautionary recommendations, such as limiting children's use of wireless devices and maintaining a safe distance from EMF-emitting sources whenever possible.

Vulnerable Populations: Children and Pregnant Women

Certain populations, such as children and pregnant women, are considered more vulnerable to the potential health effects of EMF exposure due to their developing systems and physiological differences. Understanding these vulnerabilities is crucial for implementing precautionary measures to minimise risk.

Children are more susceptible to EMF exposure for several reasons. First, their bodies are still developing, and their tissues, including the brain, are more conductive, meaning they can absorb more EMF radiation compared to adults. Children's skulls are also thinner, which allows for deeper penetration of radiofrequency (RF) radiation. This increased absorption raises concerns about potential long-term health effects, particularly with prolonged use of mobile phones and tablets. Some studies suggest that early exposure to high levels of EMF could potentially affect cognitive development and increase the risk of behavioural issues. Although these findings are not conclusive, many health authorities recommend limiting children's use of wireless devices and encouraging safe practices, such as using hands-free options.

Pregnant women are another vulnerable group. EMF exposure during pregnancy has been a topic of concern because it could potentially affect fetal development. Some studies have linked high levels of EMF exposure to an increased risk of miscarriage, preterm birth, or developmental issues in offspring. These studies suggest that the fetus may be more susceptible to EMF because of rapid cellular division and differentiation during early development. Although the evidence is not definitive, healthcare providers often recommend precautionary measures for pregnant women, such as avoiding carrying phones close to the abdomen and minimising the use of wireless devices.

Overall, while the scientific community continues to debate the exact nature of EMF's impact on vulnerable populations, adopting precautionary measures is a prudent approach to safeguard the health of children and pregnant women.

Summary: Health Effects of EMF Exposure

(a) Biological Mechanisms & Health Risks of EMF

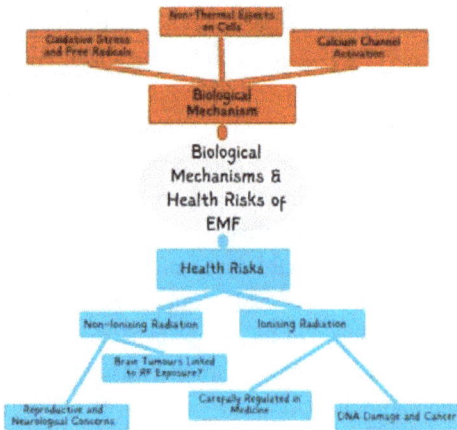

(b) Vulnerable Populations and Practical Case Study

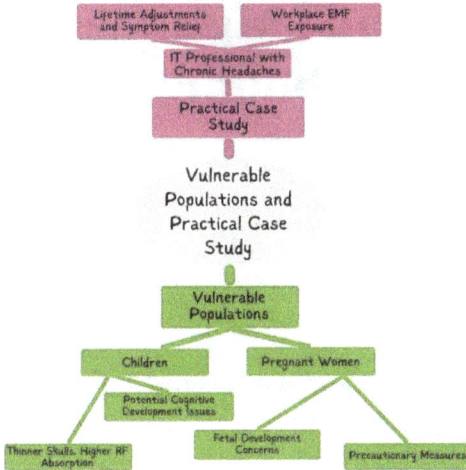

Chapter 3
Myths and Misconceptions About EMF

Common Myths About EMF

Myth 1: All EMF is Harmful

One of the most prevalent misconceptions is that **all electromagnetic fields (EMF)** are inherently harmful to human health. While it's true that certain types of EMF, like ionising radiation (X-rays, gamma rays), can pose serious health risks, this does not apply to all forms of EMF. The electromagnetic spectrum encompasses a wide range of frequencies and energy levels, from extremely low-frequency (ELF) fields emitted by power lines to high-frequency radiation like gamma rays.

Non-ionising EMFs—such as those emitted by household appliances, mobile phones, and Wi-Fi routers—do not have enough energy to ionise atoms or molecules. This means they cannot break chemical bonds in the body or directly damage DNA. Most research suggests that exposure to non-ionising EMF at typical environmental levels does not pose significant health risks.

However, this does not mean that all non-ionising EMFs are completely harmless. The concern arises with long-term, chronic exposure or when devices are used in close proximity to the body for extended periods, as these factors may have cumulative effects. For instance, using a mobile phone pressed against the ear for hours every day over many years may increase the risk of certain conditions, such as acoustic neuromas, though the evidence is not conclusive.

Therefore, while not all EMF is harmful, the context of exposure—such as duration, intensity, and distance—plays a crucial role in determining potential health effects. Distinguishing between different types of EMF and their varying levels of risk is key to understanding and addressing health concerns effectively.

Myth 2: 5G Causes Health Problems

The rollout of **5G (fifth-generation) technology** has sparked significant public debate and concern, with many people believing that 5G networks pose serious health risks. The main concern stems from the fact that 5G technology operates at higher frequencies than previous generations of wireless networks, such as 4G or 3G. These higher frequencies, often referred to as **millimetre waves**, fall within the radiofrequency (RF) spectrum, which some people fear could have more significant health effects.

However, it's important to clarify that 5G frequencies are still considered non-ionising radiation. Non-ionising radiation does not have enough energy to remove tightly bound electrons or cause ionisation, which is a key mechanism by which radiation can cause cancer and other health issues. The vast majority of scientific studies conducted on RF radiation, including frequencies used by 5G, have found no conclusive evidence that exposure to these levels of EMF causes serious health effects, such as cancer or neurological disorders.

Despite this, many myths continue to circulate, suggesting that 5G is linked to a range of health problems, including headaches, immune suppression, and even more extreme claims like causing COVID-19. These misconceptions gained traction through social media and misinformation campaigns that amplified fear and uncertainty during the pandemic. To date, no credible scientific evidence supports these claims. The World Health Organisation (WHO), International Commission on Non-Ionising Radiation Protection (ICNIRP), and numerous other health agencies have reviewed the research on 5G and have stated that exposure to 5G frequencies at typical environmental levels is unlikely to cause adverse health effects.

The fear surrounding 5G often arises from a lack of understanding of the technology and the nature of RF radiation. Millimetre waves, which are used in some 5G networks, have lower penetration depths compared to lower frequency waves. This means that they are largely absorbed by the outer layers of the skin and do not reach deeper tissues in the body. Moreover, the power output of 5G base stations and devices is strictly regulated to stay within safe exposure limits established by international health agencies.

It's also worth noting that concerns about new technologies are not unique to 5G. Each new generation of mobile networks has been met with skepticism and fear, only for subsequent research to show that they pose no significant health risks at regulated exposure levels. The same is likely true for 5G, but ongoing research will continue to monitor and evaluate potential long-term effects.

In summary, while it's important to remain vigilant and continue research, the current scientific consensus is that 5G technology is not inherently harmful to human health, and the extreme claims associated with it are not based on scientific evidence.

Myth 3: EMF Exposure Leads to Immediate Health Damage

Another common misconception is that exposure to electromagnetic fields (EMF) results in **immediate health damage** or noticeable symptoms. This myth is often propagated by anecdotal reports of individuals experiencing headaches, dizziness, or fatigue shortly after using electronic devices like cell phones or being near power lines. While these symptoms are real to the people experiencing them, scientific studies have not consistently shown that EMF exposure at typical environmental levels can cause such immediate health effects.

The perception of immediate harm is largely influenced by a phenomenon known as the **nocebo effect**. Similar to the placebo effect, where positive expectations result in perceived improvements in health, the nocebo effect occurs when negative expectations cause people to experience symptoms despite no physical cause. In the context of EMF exposure, people who are worried about potential health risks may attribute any discomfort they feel to EMF, even if the exposure levels are too low to cause harm.

Scientific research generally indicates that low-level EMF exposure does not cause acute or immediate health damage. Studies that have tested this hypothesis, including double-blind experiments where participants were unaware of their EMF exposure status, have found no consistent correlation between exposure and the onset of symptoms. For example, people who believe they are sensitive to EMF often report symptoms even when they are not actually being exposed, suggesting that psychological factors play a significant role.

This does not mean that individuals who report such symptoms should be dismissed. Instead, healthcare providers should consider the psychological and environmental factors that may be contributing to these perceptions and provide support that addresses their overall health and wellness.

Myth 4: EMF Beads and Devices Can Block Radiation

A popular misconception is that wearing **EMF-blocking devices**, such as beads, pendants, or stickers, can shield individuals from the harmful effects of electromagnetic radiation. These products are often marketed as offering protection against the radiation emitted by cell phones, Wi-Fi routers, and other electronic devices. They claim to work by blocking, absorbing, or neutralising EMF, thereby reducing exposure and mitigating health risks.

However, there is no scientific evidence to support the effectiveness of these devices. EMF is a form of electromagnetic energy, and simple objects like beads or stickers cannot alter or block the energy fields generated by electronic devices. For any object to truly shield against EMF, it would need to be made of a material capable of absorbing or reflecting electromagnetic waves, such as metal. Even then, the shielding effect is only effective if it is properly placed between the source of radiation and the person.

Many of these products are sold with exaggerated claims and lack scientific validation. Studies conducted on such devices have found that they do not significantly reduce EMF exposure levels. In some cases, the products are nothing more than decorative items with no real functionality. The marketing of these devices preys on people's fear of EMF, providing a false sense of security.

To effectively reduce EMF exposure, proven methods such as maintaining distance from sources, limiting device usage, and using grounded shielding materials (e.g., conductive fabrics or bed canopies) should be considered. Wearing beads or using stickers will not offer any measurable protection against EMF and should not be relied upon as a primary method of reducing exposure.

Myth 5: Electromagnetic Hypersensitivity is Caused by EMF

Electromagnetic hypersensitivity (EHS), also known as **Idiopathic Environmental Intolerance attributed to Electromagnetic Fields (IEI-EMF)**, is a condition where individuals report experiencing adverse health effects they believe are caused by exposure to electromagnetic fields. Symptoms often include headaches, dizziness, fatigue, skin rashes, and difficulty concentrating. People with EHS attribute these symptoms to sources such as cell phones, Wi-Fi routers, power lines, and other electronic devices.

Despite the distress experienced by those with EHS, scientific studies have not confirmed that EMF exposure is the direct cause of these symptoms. Most research indicates that the condition is not linked to the actual presence of EMF but may instead be influenced by psychological factors, such as anxiety or the nocebo effect. In controlled experiments, participants who claim to suffer from EHS often report symptoms even when they are not exposed to EMF. Conversely, they may not experience symptoms when they are unknowingly exposed to EMF, suggesting that their symptoms are not directly caused by electromagnetic fields.

The **World Health Organisation (WHO)** and other health agencies recognise EHS as a real and potentially disabling condition but classify it as a psychological or psychosomatic disorder rather than a physiological response to EMF. This does not mean that the symptoms are "all in the mind" or that they should be disregarded. On the contrary, the symptoms experienced by individuals with EHS are genuine and can significantly impact their quality of life.

Treatment for EHS typically involves managing the symptoms and addressing the psychological and environmental factors that may be contributing to the condition. Cognitive-Behavioural Therapy (CBT) has shown promise in helping individuals cope with their symptoms and reduce anxiety related to EMF exposure. Educating patients about the nature of EMF and providing reassurance can also help alleviate fears and improve outcomes.

In summary, while EHS is a real condition with genuine symptoms, current scientific evidence does not support a direct causal link between EMF exposure and the development of EHS. Addressing the condition requires a multifaceted approach that considers both psychological and environmental factors.

Psychological Effects and the Role of Media

How Media Amplifies EMF Fear

The media plays a powerful role in shaping public perception and influencing how people think about health risks associated with electromagnetic fields (EMF). Sensationalised headlines and alarming news stories can amplify fear and misinformation, leading to widespread anxiety and confusion. Media coverage often focuses on the potential dangers of new technologies, such as 5G, without providing a balanced view that includes scientific evidence or expert opinions.

One of the primary ways the media amplifies EMF fear is by highlighting individual anecdotal reports or preliminary studies that suggest a potential risk, even when these findings are not supported by the broader scientific community. For instance, a news article might feature a personal story about someone experiencing headaches or sleep disturbances due to EMF exposure from cell phones or Wi-Fi routers. Such stories, while compelling, are not representative of the general population and do not establish a causal relationship. However, when presented in a dramatic and emotional manner, they can have a strong impact on readers or viewers, making it difficult for people to differentiate between anecdotal experiences and scientifically validated evidence.

Media outlets often use fear-based language, such as "hidden dangers" or "unseen threats," to attract attention and increase viewership. This language taps into people's natural concerns about their health and safety, making the perceived threat of EMF seem more immediate and severe than it actually is. The use of scientific jargon or cherry-picking of data points without proper context can also contribute to misunderstanding. For example, the classification of radiofrequency (RF) radiation as a "possible carcinogen" by the International Agency for Research on Cancer (IARC) is often cited in media reports without explaining what this classification means. As a result, people may overestimate the actual risk posed by everyday EMF exposure.

The media's role in amplifying EMF fear has been particularly evident with the rollout of 5G technology. Conspiracy theories linking 5G to health issues like cancer, neurological disorders, and even COVID-19 have been widely circulated on social media platforms. Although these claims have been debunked by scientific experts, they have gained traction due to the viral nature of social media. People tend to share sensational content that elicits strong emotions, spreading misinformation faster than factual corrections can keep up.

Moreover, media influence can exacerbate psychological symptoms in individuals who already have health anxiety or concerns about EMF exposure. The more a person is exposed to fear-inducing information, the more likely they are to believe that EMF poses a direct threat to their health, even if their personal exposure levels are low. This can lead to a cycle of anxiety and symptom perception that reinforces their fear of EMF.

Ultimately, the media has a responsibility to report on health risks in a balanced and scientifically accurate manner. Providing context, including expert opinions, and avoiding sensationalism are essential to preventing the spread of misinformation and reducing unnecessary fear and anxiety in the public.

Understanding the Nocebo Effect

The **nocebo effect** is a psychological phenomenon where negative expectations or beliefs about a harmless substance or exposure cause individuals to experience adverse symptoms. It is the opposite of the placebo effect, where positive expectations lead to perceived improvements in health. The nocebo effect is particularly relevant in the context of electromagnetic fields (EMF) because people who are concerned about EMF exposure may experience real symptoms, even when they are not actually being exposed.

In cases of suspected electromagnetic hypersensitivity (EHS), for example, individuals often report symptoms like headaches, dizziness, fatigue, and nausea, which they believe are caused by EMF from devices like cell phones or Wi-Fi routers. However, studies have shown that these symptoms can occur even when there is no active EMF source present. In double-blind experiments, where participants are unaware of whether they are being exposed to EMF, those with self-reported EHS often experience the same symptoms whether the EMF is on or off.

The nocebo effect demonstrates the power of belief and expectation in shaping physical experiences. When people are exposed to alarming information about EMF—such as claims that it causes cancer or neurological disorders—they may become hyper-aware of any physical discomfort or health issues they experience. This heightened awareness can lead them to attribute their symptoms to EMF, even if the actual cause is unrelated. The nocebo effect can create a feedback loop where fear of EMF exposure leads to symptoms, which in turn reinforces the fear.

Understanding the nocebo effect is essential for healthcare providers working with patients who report EMF-related symptoms. Providing education, addressing fears, and promoting relaxation techniques can help alleviate symptoms and break the cycle of anxiety and symptom perception.

Summary: Myths and Misconceptions about EMF

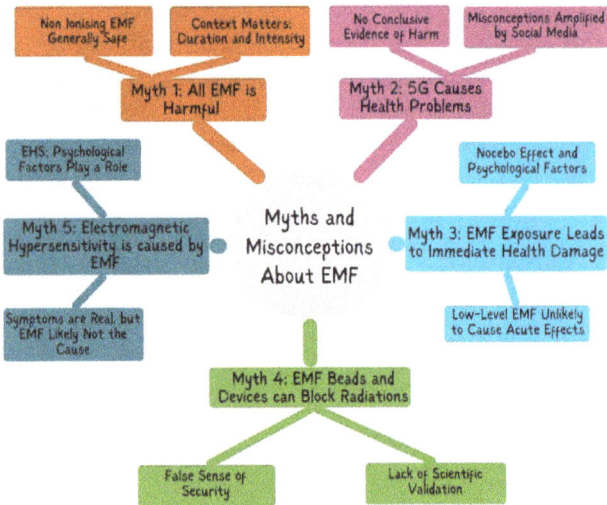

Chapter 4
Scientific Perspective vs. Conventional Thought

Interpreting EMF Risks Using Scientific Evidence

Evaluating the health risks of electromagnetic fields (EMF) requires a careful and critical approach based on scientific evidence rather than anecdotal reports or media narratives. Scientific research on EMF follows rigorous methodologies designed to minimise bias and ensure that results are reliable and replicable. This involves controlled laboratory studies, epidemiological research, and meta-analyses that combine data from multiple studies to identify overall trends and conclusions.

One of the challenges in interpreting EMF risks is that not all studies produce consistent findings. For example, some studies suggest a possible link between long-term mobile phone use and an increased risk of brain tumours, while others find no significant association. These discrepancies can arise due to differences in study design, sample size, exposure assessment, and confounding factors such as genetics, lifestyle, and environmental influences. To address these issues, scientific consensus is built through comprehensive reviews and evaluations by expert panels, such as the International Commission on Non-Ionising Radiation Protection (ICNIRP) and the World Health Organisation (WHO).

When assessing EMF risks, it is essential to distinguish between **statistical association** and **causation**. Just because a study finds an association between EMF exposure and a health outcome does not mean that EMF directly caused the outcome. Establishing causation requires demonstrating a clear mechanism by which EMF exposure leads to specific biological changes that result in disease. For most non-ionising EMF, such a mechanism has not been conclusively identified.

Moreover, scientific evidence must consider the context of exposure. Many laboratory studies use EMF levels that are far higher than what people typically encounter in their daily lives. While these studies can provide insights into potential mechanisms of action, their findings may not be applicable to real-world situations. Therefore, regulatory agencies set exposure limits based on both experimental data and real-world exposure levels to ensure public safety.

Scientific evidence also evolves over time as new technologies and research methods become available. For example, the transition from 4G to 5G has prompted new studies on the health effects of millimetre waves, which were not previously used in widespread consumer applications. Ongoing research helps to refine our understanding of EMF risks and guide public health recommendations.

In summary, interpreting EMF risks using scientific evidence involves weighing the totality of research, understanding study limitations, and distinguishing between association and causation. This evidence-based approach provides a more accurate and balanced perspective than relying on media reports or personal anecdotes.

Understanding Gaps in Long-term Research

Despite decades of research on the health effects of electromagnetic fields (EMF), several gaps in knowledge remain, particularly regarding the long-term impacts of chronic, low-level exposure. These gaps exist for various reasons, including the evolving nature of technology, the difficulty of measuring long-term exposure, and ethical considerations that limit experimental research on humans.

One of the primary challenges in studying the long-term effects of EMF is the rapid pace of technological change. As new technologies like 5G are introduced, the nature of EMF exposure changes, making it difficult to conduct long-term studies that keep pace with these advancements. For instance, the widespread use of mobile phones began in the 1990s, and many studies on mobile phone radiation have only followed participants for a decade or less. The full health impact of mobile phone use may not be apparent for another 10-20 years, especially if there are delayed effects that take decades to manifest.

Additionally, accurately assessing long-term EMF exposure is challenging. Many studies rely on self-reported data, such as the frequency and duration of mobile phone use, which can be subject to recall bias. Moreover, individuals are often exposed to multiple sources of EMF in varying intensities throughout the day, making it difficult to isolate the effects of a single source. The development of wearable devices that measure real-time exposure may help improve future research, but these tools are not yet widely used in epidemiological studies.

Ethical considerations also limit experimental research on humans. Exposing people to potentially harmful levels of EMF for extended periods would be unethical, so researchers must rely on observational studies that track individuals' health outcomes over time. These studies are valuable, but they cannot establish causation as effectively as randomised controlled trials.

Another gap in research is the limited focus on vulnerable populations, such as children and pregnant women. While some studies have explored the effects of EMF on these groups, more research is needed to understand how developmental stages or physiological differences may alter susceptibility to EMF exposure.

Finally, the potential for cumulative effects of EMF exposure has not been thoroughly investigated. Many studies examine a single type of exposure, such as RF from cell phones, without considering how simultaneous exposure to other sources (e.g., Wi-Fi, Bluetooth, power lines) might interact to influence health outcomes. Addressing these gaps will require collaboration across disciplines, the development of new research tools, and long-term studies that follow participants for decades.

Differentiating Real Risks from Myths

Differentiating between real risks and myths surrounding electromagnetic fields (EMF) is essential for making informed decisions about health and safety. This process involves critically evaluating the available scientific evidence, understanding the limitations of studies, and recognising the role of misinformation in shaping public perception.

One of the first steps in distinguishing real risks from myths is to understand the **types of studies** that provide reliable evidence. Randomised controlled trials (RCTs) and well-conducted epidemiological studies offer higher levels of evidence compared to anecdotal reports or case studies. Meta-analyses and systematic reviews, which aggregate findings from multiple studies, provide a more comprehensive picture of the evidence and can help identify consistent trends or areas of uncertainty.

It is also important to consider the **dose-response relationship** when evaluating EMF risks. For example, high levels of ionising radiation are known to cause cancer, but low-level non-ionising radiation, such as that emitted by Wi-Fi routers, has not been shown to have the same effect. Understanding the intensity and duration of exposure is crucial for assessing risk. Exposures that are minimal or infrequent are unlikely to pose significant health risks, whereas long-term, high-level exposure may warrant precautionary measures.

Additionally, many myths arise from **misinterpretations of scientific terminology**. Terms like "possible carcinogen" or "association" can be easily misunderstood by the public, leading to exaggerated perceptions of risk. Clarifying what these terms mean in a scientific context helps to mitigate unnecessary fear and anxiety.

Finally, the influence of **misinformation and conspiracy theories** should not be underestimated. False claims that link 5G technology to COVID-19, for example, can spread rapidly on social media, creating widespread fear despite a lack of scientific basis. Combatting these myths requires transparent communication, accessible education, and engagement with trusted sources of information.

In conclusion, differentiating real risks from myths involves critical thinking, a solid understanding of scientific evidence, and the ability to discern credible sources from those that promote fear and misinformation.

Clinical Case Study: 45-year-old Woman with Electromagnetic Hypersensitivity (EHS)

Case Introduction and Patient Profile

The patient is a 45-year-old woman who reports experiencing a range of distressing symptoms that she believes are caused by exposure to electromagnetic fields (EMF). Her symptoms began approximately two years ago and include chronic headaches, severe fatigue, skin rashes, and insomnia. The patient has since made significant lifestyle changes to avoid EMF, including moving her bed away from power outlets, switching off her home's Wi-Fi, and minimising her use of electronic devices. Despite these measures, her symptoms persist, leading to increased anxiety and social isolation.

The patient describes herself as otherwise healthy, with no history of chronic medical conditions or mental health disorders. She works as an accountant, which requires prolonged use of computers and smartphones. Although her symptoms improve slightly on weekends when she spends time outdoors, they return as soon as she resumes her regular work routine. Concerned that her symptoms are disrupting her quality of life, she seeks medical advice to address her perceived EMF sensitivity.

Symptoms and Evaluation

The patient's primary symptoms include persistent headaches, fatigue, dizziness, nausea, insomnia, and a sensation of tingling or burning on her skin. She reports that these symptoms intensify when she is near sources of EMF, such as Wi-Fi routers, cell phones, and other electronic devices. She has avoided using her mobile phone for calls, opting to communicate through text messages instead. She also experiences a sense of discomfort and anxiety when entering places with visible electronic equipment, such as offices or coffee shops.

During the initial evaluation, a comprehensive medical history and physical examination are conducted. Neurological and dermatological exams reveal no abnormalities, and her lab tests, including blood work, thyroid function, and electrolyte levels, are all within normal ranges. Imaging studies, including an MRI of the brain, show no structural abnormalities that could explain her symptoms.

The patient is referred for a psychological assessment to evaluate the potential role of psychological factors in her condition. The results suggest that her symptoms are not directly caused by physiological changes in response to EMF but may be influenced by heightened anxiety and a fear of EMF exposure. The evaluation highlights the presence of health anxiety and a strong nocebo response, where negative expectations and beliefs about EMF exposure exacerbate her symptoms. Based on these findings, the diagnosis of **Electromagnetic Hypersensitivity (EHS)** is considered, with the understanding that the symptoms are real but not directly caused by EMF exposure.

Interventions and Outcome

Given the complex nature of her symptoms and the impact on her quality of life, a multidisciplinary approach is recommended. The patient is advised to participate in **cognitive-behavioural therapy (CBT)** to address her anxiety and modify her negative beliefs about EMF. CBT sessions focus on helping her identify and challenge distorted thoughts related to EMF exposure, gradually increasing her comfort around electronic devices through controlled exposure therapy and teaching her relaxation techniques to manage stress.

Additionally, she is introduced to **mindfulness-based stress reduction (MBSR)**, which includes breathing exercises, meditation, and progressive muscle relaxation, to reduce her overall anxiety and improve her ability to cope with perceived EMF-related symptoms. As part of her treatment plan, she is encouraged to limit her consumption of media that discusses EMF risks, as these sources have been contributing to her fear and anxiety. Instead, she is provided with educational materials that present balanced, evidence-based information on EMF.

Over the course of three months, the patient reports a gradual reduction in symptom severity and frequency. Her headaches become less frequent, and she no longer experiences skin tingling. She is able to use her computer for longer periods without discomfort and has resumed making short phone calls. Although she still experiences mild anxiety in highly "connected" environments, she feels more in control and less fearful. The integration of CBT, MBSR, and educational support has significantly improved her quality of life and reduced the impact of EHS on her daily activities.

Summary: Scientific Perspective vs Conventional Thought

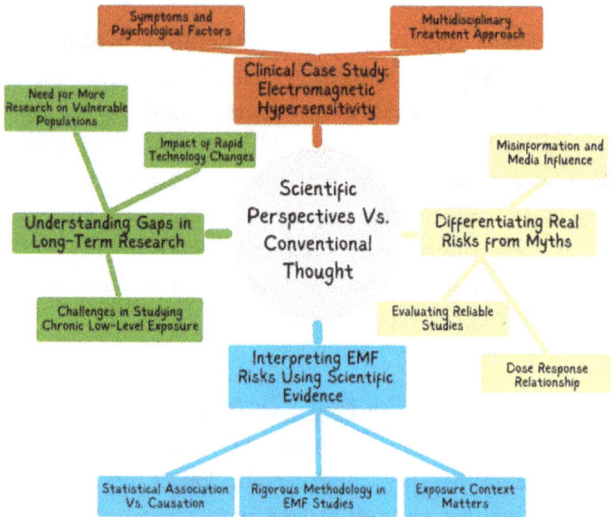

Chapter 5
Practical Ways to Reduce
EMF Exposure

Reducing EMF exposure involves a combination of lifestyle changes, behaviour modifications, and the use of specialised products to minimise exposure to electromagnetic fields. This section outlines practical strategies to reduce EMF exposure in the home and workplace, helping to create a healthier environment without sacrificing the benefits of modern technology.

Reducing EMF Exposure at Home

Turning Off Wi-Fi at Night

One of the simplest and most effective ways to reduce EMF exposure at home is to turn off your Wi-Fi router at night. Wi-Fi routers emit constant radiofrequency (RF) radiation, even when no devices are connected. During sleep, the body is more vulnerable to environmental factors, and minimising exposure to RF radiation can support better rest and overall health.

Turning off the Wi-Fi at night eliminates unnecessary radiation when the network is not in use. This can be done manually or using an automatic timer that turns off the router at a specified time and restarts it in the morning. Alternatively, consider switching to a wired Ethernet connection, which provides a reliable and faster internet connection without emitting RF radiation.

For families with young children, turning off the Wi-Fi at night is particularly beneficial, as children's developing systems are more sensitive to environmental factors like EMF. It is also a simple way to instill good habits around the use of technology and promote better sleep hygiene. Beyond health benefits, turning off the Wi-Fi at night can also lead to energy savings and a reduced carbon footprint.

Incorporating this change into your routine is straightforward and cost-effective, making it an excellent starting point for reducing EMF exposure at home.

Using Wired Connections Instead of Wi-Fi

Using wired connections, such as Ethernet cables, instead of Wi-Fi is another effective strategy for reducing RF radiation exposure. Wi-Fi routers continuously emit RF radiation to maintain a wireless network connection, even when devices are not actively transmitting data. By switching to wired connections, you can eliminate this source of radiation and create a safer environment, particularly in areas where people spend extended periods, such as bedrooms, home offices, and living rooms.

Setting up a wired network involves connecting devices like computers, gaming consoles, and smart TVs directly to the router using Ethernet cables. This not only reduces RF exposure but also offers a more secure and stable internet connection. For devices that cannot be connected via Ethernet, consider using powerline adapters, which transmit the internet signal through the home's electrical wiring, providing a wired connection without additional cabling.

For households with multiple devices, adopting a mixed approach can be beneficial. Keep essential devices like desktop computers and smart TVs on wired connections, and limit Wi-Fi usage to portable devices like smartphones and tablets. Additionally, most modern routers allow you to lower the power output of the Wi-Fi signal or schedule specific times for the Wi-Fi to be turned on and off, which can further reduce RF exposure.

Switching to wired connections might require some initial setup and adjustment but offers long-term benefits in terms of reduced RF radiation, improved internet performance, and enhanced security. This strategy is particularly useful for individuals who are sensitive to EMF or want to create a safer environment for children and family members.

Keeping Devices at a Safe Distance

Maintaining a safe distance from electronic devices is one of the easiest and most effective ways to reduce EMF exposure. The strength of electromagnetic radiation decreases exponentially with distance, meaning that even a small increase in distance can significantly lower exposure levels. This principle applies to all devices that emit EMF, including mobile phones, tablets, laptops, and Wi-Fi routers.

For mobile phones, using the speakerphone function or wired earphones instead of holding the phone directly against the ear reduces exposure to RF radiation. Additionally, avoiding carrying the phone in a pocket or close to the body when not in use can further reduce exposure. Consider placing the phone on a desk or table instead of carrying it on your person, and keep it in aeroplane mode when not actively needed.

Laptops and tablets should not be placed directly on the lap for extended periods. Instead, use a desk or table to create distance between the device and your body. Using external keyboards and mice can also increase the distance between you and the device, minimising exposure.

Wi-Fi routers should be positioned away from frequently used spaces, such as living rooms and bedrooms. Place them in less frequently occupied areas, like a hallway or a dedicated office, and keep them elevated to maximise signal strength while reducing exposure.

Creating distance between yourself and EMF-emitting devices is a simple yet powerful way to minimise exposure. Encouraging these practices at home and work can significantly reduce overall EMF exposure and promote a healthier environment.

Moving Large Appliances Away from Living Spaces

Large appliances, such as refrigerators, washing machines, and microwaves, are often significant sources of EMF in the home. These appliances emit extremely low-frequency (ELF) radiation, which is most intense close to the appliance and diminishes rapidly with distance. Placing these appliances thoughtfully can help reduce overall EMF exposure, especially in small living spaces.

Refrigerators, for instance, should be positioned away from areas where people spend a lot of time, such as dining tables or seating areas. If possible, place the refrigerator against an external wall to prevent ELF radiation from penetrating deeper into living spaces. Similarly, washing machines, dryers, and other laundry equipment should be placed in a separate laundry room or utility area, reducing the likelihood of prolonged exposure when these appliances are in use.

Microwaves are a unique concern because they emit both ELF and RF radiation. Modern microwaves are designed to limit radiation leakage, but standing close to them while they are operating can increase exposure. It's advisable to stand at least a few feet away from the microwave when it's in use and avoid placing it near frequently used countertops or seating areas.

For homes with open floor plans, where it may be difficult to separate appliances from living areas, consider using shielding materials. Conductive shielding fabrics or paints can be applied to walls adjacent to high-EMF appliances to reduce radiation levels. Additionally, using timers or smart plugs to control when these appliances are active can further minimise unnecessary exposure.

By moving large appliances away from living spaces, you can reduce both ELF and RF radiation exposure in the home, contributing to a healthier and safer environment.

Creating an EMF-Free Sleeping Environment

Creating an EMF-free or low-EMF sleeping environment is essential because sleep is a critical time for the body to rest and repair. Exposure to EMF during sleep can disrupt melatonin production, a hormone that regulates sleep and has antioxidant properties. This disruption can lead to poor sleep quality, insomnia, and potentially long-term health issues. Reducing EMF exposure in the bedroom can improve sleep quality and overall health.

To create an EMF-free sleeping environment, start by removing electronic devices from the bedroom. Mobile phones, tablets, and laptops should be turned off or placed in another room. If you need to keep your phone in the bedroom for emergencies, set it to aeroplane mode and keep it at least six feet away from the bed. Replacing a smartphone alarm with a traditional alarm clock can help reduce the temptation to keep electronic devices nearby.

Turn off or unplug non-essential electronics, such as televisions and Wi-Fi routers. If turning off the Wi-Fi router is not feasible, consider placing it as far away from the bedroom as possible or using a timer to automatically turn it off during sleep hours.

Minimise electrical wiring near the bed. Avoid placing the bed against walls with significant electrical wiring or outlets, as these can emit ELF radiation. If rewiring is not feasible, consider using EMF-blocking materials, such as shielding paint or fabrics, to create a protective barrier around the bed. Shielding can also be used on windows to reduce RF radiation from external sources like cell towers.

For individuals who are particularly sensitive to EMF, grounding techniques such as using earthing mats or sheets may help. These products connect to the Earth's natural electrical field, promoting relaxation and potentially counteracting the effects of low-level EMF exposure.

Using an EMF meter to measure radiation levels before and after implementing changes can help identify hidden EMF sources and ensure that the modifications are effective. Creating an EMF-free sleeping environment can significantly improve sleep quality, support overall health, and reduce long-term exposure to electromagnetic radiation.

Reducing EMF Exposure at Work

Taking Regular Breaks from Screens

Taking regular breaks from screens and electronic devices is essential for reducing EMF exposure in the workplace. Prolonged use of computers, tablets, and smartphones increases exposure to low-level EMF and can contribute to eye strain, mental fatigue, and musculoskeletal discomfort. Incorporating breaks into your routine can mitigate these effects and promote better health and wellness.

The **20-20-20 rule** is a simple guideline: every 20 minutes, look at something 20 feet away for 20 seconds. This helps to reduce eye strain and provides a brief respite from screen exposure. Standing up, stretching, and moving around every hour can also help alleviate the physical strain associated with long periods of sitting and working on electronic devices.

Using ergonomic workstations and positioning electronic devices to maintain a comfortable distance can also reduce EMF exposure. For instance, placing monitors at least 20 inches away from the eyes and positioning keyboards at a comfortable height can improve posture and reduce strain.

Regular breaks, combined with ergonomic adjustments and strategic device placement, can create a healthier work environment and minimise the impact of prolonged EMF exposure.

Avoiding Prolonged Use of Bluetooth and Wireless Devices

Bluetooth devices, such as wireless earbuds, keyboards, and mice, emit RF radiation similar to that of Wi-Fi and mobile phones. While the levels are generally lower, prolonged use can contribute to overall EMF exposure. Reducing the use of these devices, especially when there are wired alternatives available, is a practical way to lower exposure.

For instance, using wired earphones instead of wireless earbuds reduces direct RF exposure near the head. Similarly, opting for wired keyboards and mice instead of Bluetooth versions minimises RF emissions near your hands and body. In environments where multiple Bluetooth devices are active, such as open-plan offices, cumulative exposure can be higher. Reducing the number of active wireless connections and using wired alternatives where feasible can help create a healthier work environment.

If wireless devices are necessary, consider using them for short durations and switching to wired options whenever possible. Limiting the use of Bluetooth and other wireless devices is especially important for individuals who are sensitive to EMF or wish to reduce their overall exposure as a precautionary measure.

Using EMF Shielding Products

EMF shielding products are designed to block or redirect electromagnetic radiation, reducing exposure levels in specific areas. These products include shielding fabrics, paints, bed canopies, window films, and clothing made from materials that contain conductive metals like silver or copper, which reflect or absorb EMF.

Shielding Fabrics and Bed Canopies: Shielding fabrics can be used to create EMF-reducing curtains, bedding, and clothing. Bed canopies made from these fabrics are particularly effective for creating low-EMF sleeping areas. The canopies are draped over the bed to block RF radiation from external sources like cell towers or Wi-Fi routers, offering a protected space for rest.

Shielding Paints: Shielding paints contain conductive particles that absorb and block both RF and ELF radiation. They can be applied to walls, ceilings, and floors to create a shielded space, reducing EMF penetration from outside sources. When using shielding paints, it's crucial to ground the painted surfaces properly to ensure that the shield functions correctly.

Window Films and Protective Clothing: EMF-blocking window films can reduce radiation penetration through windows, which is especially useful for homes or offices near cell towers or power lines. Protective clothing made from EMF-shielding materials offers portable protection, particularly for individuals who are sensitive to EMF.

While shielding products can significantly reduce EMF exposure, they should be used as part of a broader strategy that includes behavioural changes and device management. Measuring EMF levels before and after installing shielding products is recommended to ensure they are effective and to identify any potential hotspots created by improper installation.

Products and Tools for EMF Reduction

EMF reduction tools can be an effective way to create a safer and healthier environment at home or in the workplace. These products range from shielding materials that block electromagnetic radiation to grounding devices that help neutralise EMF effects. While no single product can entirely eliminate exposure, when used in combination with lifestyle changes, these tools can significantly reduce EMF levels.

Bed Canopies, Curtains, and Shielding Paints (400 words)

Bed canopies, shielding curtains, and EMF-blocking paints are some of the most powerful tools for reducing exposure to electromagnetic fields (EMF) in specific areas, such as bedrooms or home offices. These products work by creating a barrier that blocks or reflects electromagnetic radiation, providing a protected space that is shielded from external and internal sources of EMF.

1. **Bed Canopies**: Made from conductive materials like silver or copper, bed canopies are designed to form a Faraday cage around the bed. This setup significantly reduces radiofrequency (RF) exposure from nearby cell towers, Wi-Fi routers, and other sources. Bed canopies are especially beneficial for individuals with electromagnetic hypersensitivity (EHS) or those living near high-EMF sources. To use a bed canopy effectively, it should be grounded and securely draped around the bed, ensuring that all sides are covered.

2. **Shielding Curtains**: Similar to bed canopies, shielding curtains are made from conductive fabrics that block RF radiation. These curtains can be used on windows and doors to prevent EMF penetration from outside sources like cell towers or neighbors' Wi-Fi signals. Shielding curtains are a practical option for reducing EMF in living spaces, particularly in urban areas with high levels of ambient radiation.

3. **Shielding Paints**: Shielding paints are infused with conductive particles that block both RF and extremely low-frequency (ELF) radiation. These paints are applied to walls, ceilings, and floors to create a shielded space. Shielding paints are particularly effective in homes or offices located near power lines or mobile phone towers. However, it is essential to ground the painted surfaces properly to ensure that they effectively block radiation and do not create unintended hotspots.

While these products can significantly reduce EMF exposure, they should be part of a comprehensive strategy that includes other methods like turning off devices when not in use, maintaining distance, and limiting usage. Measuring EMF levels before and after installation can help confirm that the shielding is effective.

Phone and Laptop Cases

EMF-blocking phone and laptop cases are designed to reduce exposure to radiation emitted by these devices. These cases typically use layers of conductive materials, such as copper or silver, which absorb or reflect RF radiation away from the body. While they can be effective in reducing direct exposure, it is important to use these cases correctly to avoid inadvertently increasing radiation levels.

1. **Phone Cases**: EMF-blocking phone cases are often equipped with a shielding layer on the front cover. When closed, the case can reduce exposure to RF radiation during calls or while carrying the phone in a pocket. However, it's crucial to ensure that the case does not block the phone's signal, as this can cause the device to increase its power output, potentially raising overall radiation levels. For best results, use the phone in speaker mode or with wired earphones, and keep the phone away from the body as much as possible.
2. **Laptop Cases and Pads**: Laptop shielding cases and pads are placed between the laptop and the user's body to block RF and ELF radiation emitted from the device. These pads are particularly useful for reducing exposure during prolonged use, especially when the laptop is placed on the lap. Some cases also have built-in heat shields, offering added comfort and safety.

While EMF-blocking cases can reduce exposure to a certain extent, they should be used in conjunction with other practices, such as keeping devices at a distance and turning off wireless functions when not needed. These cases are not a substitute for comprehensive EMF reduction strategies but can complement other efforts to lower exposure.

Grounding Mats and Sheets

Grounding mats and sheets, also known as earthing products, connect the body to the Earth's natural electric field, which can help neutralise free radicals and reduce the impact of low-level EMF exposure. These products are typically made with conductive materials like carbon or silver, which facilitate the transfer of electrons from the Earth into the body, promoting relaxation and potentially alleviating symptoms associated with EMF sensitivity.

1. **Grounding Mats**: Grounding mats are commonly used under desks, on beds, or in areas where people spend long periods, such as workstations or relaxation zones. They are connected to a grounded outlet or directly to the Earth using a grounding rod. The theory behind grounding is that it helps to equalise the body's electrical potential with that of the Earth, reducing the effects of ambient EMF exposure.
2. **Grounding Sheets**: Grounding sheets are used on beds, providing a grounded surface for the body during sleep. They are particularly beneficial for individuals who experience sleep disturbances or anxiety related to EMF exposure. To use grounding sheets effectively, they must be in contact with bare skin and connected to a proper grounding source.

Although research on grounding is still emerging, some studies suggest that it can improve sleep quality, reduce inflammation, and promote overall health and wellness. Grounding products should be used alongside other EMF reduction strategies, as they do not block RF or ELF radiation but may offer complementary benefits by promoting relaxation and reducing oxidative stress.

Clinical Case Study: Family Reducing EMF for Better Sleep

Case Introduction and Family Profile

The case involves a family of four—parents and two children aged 8 and 10—who have been experiencing sleep disturbances and behavioural changes over the past year. The parents reported that both children frequently wake up during the night and struggle to fall back asleep. The family lives in a high-density urban area surrounded by multiple cell towers and has numerous electronic devices in the home, including Wi-Fi routers, smart TVs, and tablets.

Concerned about the potential impact of electromagnetic fields (EMF) on their health, the parents sought professional guidance on creating a low-EMF environment, particularly in the children's bedrooms. The goal was to improve sleep quality and overall health and wellness by reducing EMF exposure at night.

Symptoms and Evaluation

The family reported that the children had difficulty falling asleep, often waking up multiple times during the night with complaints of headaches and feeling anxious. During the day, the children showed signs of irritability and reduced focus, which affected their school performance and social interactions.

An initial EMF assessment was conducted in the home, revealing high levels of radiofrequency (RF) radiation in the children's bedrooms, mainly due to the proximity of the Wi-Fi router and the use of tablets close to bedtime. Elevated levels of extremely low-frequency (ELF) radiation were also detected from electrical wiring near the headboards of the children's beds. Based on these findings, it was recommended that the family take immediate steps to reduce EMF exposure, particularly during the night when the children were most affected.

The family was advised to turn off the Wi-Fi router at night, move the children's beds away from walls with significant electrical wiring, and implement the use of EMF-shielding bed canopies to create a protected sleeping area. These changes were expected to reduce overall exposure and promote better sleep quality.

Interventions and Outcome

The family implemented several interventions over a month. First, they began turning off the Wi-Fi router at night and limited screen time in the evening. All electronic devices, including tablets and phones, were removed from the children's bedrooms before bedtime. The children's beds were also moved away from walls with significant electrical wiring, and the family purchased EMF-shielding bed canopies made from conductive fabric, which were installed over the children's beds.

Within a few weeks, the family noticed positive changes. The children reported falling asleep more quickly and staying asleep throughout the night. Their morning headaches disappeared, and they appeared more energetic and focused during the day. The parents also observed an improvement in the children's mood and behaviour, with less irritability and better concentration at school.

A follow-up EMF assessment showed a significant reduction in RF and ELF radiation levels in the children's bedrooms. The parents expressed satisfaction with the results and felt that the changes had contributed to a healthier and more restful environment for the entire family. Although it is difficult to attribute the improvements solely to EMF reduction, the overall positive outcome suggests that minimising exposure played a role in enhancing sleep quality and health and wellness.

This case study highlights the importance of creating a low-EMF environment, especially for children who may be more sensitive to the effects of prolonged exposure. Practical interventions, such as turning off Wi-Fi, using shielding products, and modifying the layout of living spaces, can lead to meaningful improvements in health and quality of life.

Creating an Action Plan

Checklist for Reducing EMF Exposure

1. **Turn Off Wi-Fi When Not in Use**: Disable your Wi-Fi router at night or when it is not needed to reduce RF radiation exposure.
2. **Use Wired Connections**: Opt for Ethernet cables for devices like computers, gaming consoles, and smart TVs instead of relying on Wi-Fi.
3. **Keep Devices at a Distance**: Maintain a safe distance from EMF-emitting devices. Avoid carrying your phone in your pocket or holding it close to your head during calls.
4. **Limit Bluetooth and Wireless Device Use**: Use wired options whenever possible, such as earphones or keyboards, to minimise RF exposure.
5. **Create an EMF-Free Sleeping Environment**: Remove electronic devices from bedrooms, turn off Wi-Fi at night, and use shielding products like bed canopies or curtains.
6. **Reposition Large Appliances**: Place refrigerators, washing machines, and microwaves away from frequently occupied areas.
7. **Measure EMF Levels**: Use an EMF metre to identify high-EMF areas in your home and take appropriate measures to reduce exposure.
8. **Use Shielding Products**: Consider using EMF-blocking paints, fabrics, or bed canopies to create low-EMF zones.
9. **Implement Grounding Techniques**: Use grounding mats or sheets to connect with the Earth's natural energy, promoting relaxation and potentially counteracting EMF effects.
10. **Educate and Stay Informed**: Keep up-to-date with the latest research on EMF and incorporate new findings into your exposure reduction strategies.

Combining Strategies for Maximum Benefit

Combining multiple EMF reduction strategies creates a comprehensive approach that maximises protection and promotes a healthier living environment. No single product or intervention can entirely eliminate EMF exposure, but integrating several practices can significantly reduce overall exposure levels.

For example, turning off the Wi-Fi router at night, using wired connections, and creating distance from devices can reduce RF radiation. Adding shielding products, such as bed canopies or paints, can further block external sources of EMF, while grounding techniques provide additional health benefits. Implementing these strategies together addresses various sources of EMF and offers a more holistic approach to managing exposure.

It is also essential to monitor the effectiveness of these interventions using an EMF meter. Regular measurements can help identify areas where additional actions are needed and ensure that shielding products are working as intended. Adjusting the position of devices, changing the layout of furniture, and modifying daily habits can have a significant cumulative effect in reducing exposure.

Finally, fostering awareness and encouraging family members to participate in EMF reduction practices can create a more cohesive effort. Educating children and other household members about the benefits of minimising EMF exposure and using devices responsibly can lead to lasting habits that promote overall health and wellness.

Summary: Practical Ways to Reduce EMF Exposure

(a) Reducing EMF Exposure at Home

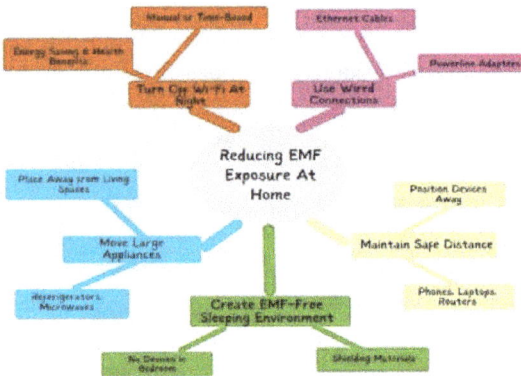

(b) Reducing EMF Exposure at Work

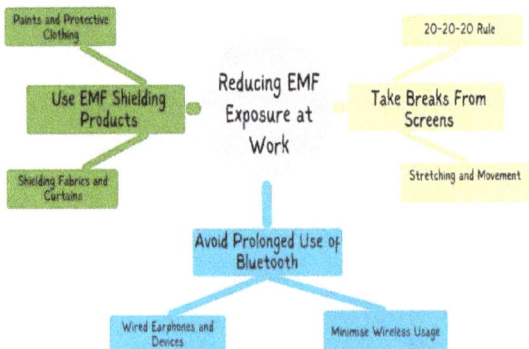

Chapter 6
Introduction to Earthing

Historical Background and Definition

The concept of earthing is not new; it has roots in the natural lifestyles of our ancestors, who were in constant contact with the Earth's surface. Historically, humans walked barefoot, slept on the ground, and used natural materials in their dwellings, which provided a continuous connection to the Earth's natural electric field. This connection is believed to have supported overall health and health and wellness by maintaining the body's bioelectrical balance.

With the advent of modern living, our lifestyles have changed dramatically. People now wear rubber-soled shoes, live in insulated homes, and are surrounded by synthetic materials that isolate them from the Earth's energy. This disconnection, along with the rise in EMF exposure from electronic devices, has been suggested as a contributing factor to various health issues, including increased inflammation, stress, and sleep disturbances.

The practice of earthing, or grounding, aims to reconnect the body with the Earth's natural electric field by walking barefoot on natural surfaces such as grass, sand, or soil, or by using grounding products like mats and sheets indoors. The idea is that direct contact with the Earth allows electrons to flow from the ground into the body, neutralising free radicals and reducing oxidative stress. While this concept may seem unconventional, emerging scientific research suggests that earthing may have measurable physiological benefits.

In essence, earthing is a return to a more natural way of living that aligns with the human body's evolutionary history. It seeks to restore the body's natural electrical balance, which may be disrupted by modern lifestyles and environmental factors, such as EMF exposure.

The Concept of Connecting to the Earth's Energy

Earthing is based on the principle that the Earth's surface is electrically conductive and possesses a natural electric field. This field is rich in free electrons, which are negatively charged particles that can flow into the body when there is direct contact with the ground. The concept is rooted in the understanding that the human body is also electrically conductive, and regular contact with the Earth's energy helps maintain the body's electrical stability and homeostasis.

Proponents of earthing suggest that this flow of electrons into the body helps neutralise positively charged free radicals, which are produced during normal metabolic processes and in response to environmental stressors, such as exposure to electromagnetic fields (EMF). Free radicals are highly reactive molecules that can cause oxidative damage to cells and contribute to inflammation and chronic disease. By providing a source of free electrons, earthing is thought to counteract the effects of oxidative stress, thereby reducing inflammation and promoting overall health.

The concept of connecting to the Earth's energy is supported by the observation that many physiological processes in the body are influenced by electrical charges and fields. For example, the heart, brain, and nervous system all function through the generation and conduction of electrical impulses. Disruptions to the body's electrical environment, such as through chronic EMF exposure, can potentially interfere with these processes, leading to imbalances and health issues.

Earthing seeks to reestablish the body's natural electrical connection with the Earth, thereby stabilising its bioelectrical environment. This can lead to improved cellular function, enhanced immune response, and better regulation of circadian rhythms. While more research is needed to fully understand the mechanisms behind earthing, the concept offers a plausible explanation for how reconnecting with the Earth's energy could support health and health and wellness.

Scientific Research on Earthing

Overview of Existing Studies

Research on earthing is still in its early stages, but existing studies suggest that grounding can have a range of positive health effects. The majority of research has focused on earthing's impact on inflammation, stress, and sleep quality, as well as its potential role in reducing symptoms associated with chronic diseases.

One of the earliest studies on earthing, published in 2004 in the *Journal of Alternative and Complementary Medicine*, found that grounding the body during sleep by using an earthing mat reduced cortisol levels and improved sleep quality in participants. Cortisol is a hormone associated with the body's stress response, and its regulation is critical for maintaining a healthy sleep-wake cycle. This study suggested that grounding could help modulate the body's stress response, leading to better sleep and overall health.

Subsequent research has explored earthing's effects on inflammation. A 2010 study published in the *Journal of Environmental and Public Health* demonstrated that grounding significantly reduced markers of inflammation in subjects after physical exercise. Participants who used grounding techniques showed less muscle damage and faster recovery times, indicating that earthing could play a role in mitigating exercise-induced inflammation and accelerating healing.

Another area of research has focused on earthing's impact on cardiovascular health. A 2013 study found that earthing improved blood flow and reduced blood viscosity, which are critical factors in cardiovascular health. Improved blood flow can enhance oxygen delivery to tissues and reduce the risk of clot formation, potentially lowering the risk of heart disease.

While these studies are promising, it is important to note that much of the research on earthing has been conducted on small sample sizes, and more extensive, randomised controlled trials are needed to confirm these findings. Additionally, the mechanisms by which earthing exerts its effects are not yet fully understood, making it a subject of ongoing scientific inquiry.

Overall, existing studies suggest that earthing may offer a range of health benefits, particularly in reducing inflammation, modulating stress responses, and improving sleep quality. However, further research is needed to establish definitive conclusions and explore additional health outcomes.

1. *Effects on Inflammation*

Inflammation is the body's natural response to injury or infection, but chronic inflammation can contribute to a range of health problems, including cardiovascular disease, diabetes, and autoimmune disorders. Earthing is believed to reduce inflammation by promoting the transfer of free electrons from the Earth into the body, which neutralises positively charged free radicals and reduces oxidative stress.

Research has shown that grounding can lower levels of inflammatory markers in the body. In a study conducted by Chevalier et al. (2010), participants who used grounding techniques after engaging in strenuous physical activity experienced reduced levels of C-reactive protein (CRP), a key marker of inflammation. Additionally, thermographic imaging, which detects heat patterns associated with inflammation, showed significant reductions in inflammation in grounded subjects compared to those who were not grounded.

These findings suggest that earthing may be particularly beneficial for individuals with chronic inflammatory conditions, such as arthritis or fibromyalgia. By reducing inflammation, earthing could potentially alleviate pain, improve mobility, and enhance overall quality of life. However, more research is needed to confirm these effects and understand the underlying mechanisms.

2. *Effects on Stress and Anxiety*

Stress and anxiety are common issues that can significantly impact quality of life. Chronic stress is associated with an increased risk of various health problems, including cardiovascular disease, digestive disorders, and mental health conditions. Earthing has been proposed as a natural way to reduce stress and anxiety by stabilising the body's autonomic nervous system and promoting relaxation.

Studies have shown that earthing can influence heart rate variability (HRV), a measure of autonomic nervous system function. Higher HRV is associated with better stress resilience and a greater ability to adapt to environmental changes. In a study published in *Integrative Medicine: A Clinician's Journal*, participants who practised earthing had higher HRV compared to those who did not, indicating reduced stress levels and improved autonomic function.

Another study examined the effects of earthing on cortisol, the body's primary stress hormone. Cortisol levels typically follow a diurnal rhythm, peaking in the morning and gradually decreasing throughout the day. Dysregulated cortisol rhythms are associated with chronic stress, insomnia, and anxiety. The study found that grounding during sleep normalised cortisol levels and improved overall stress responses in participants.

These findings suggest that earthing can have a calming effect on the nervous system, helping to alleviate symptoms of stress and anxiety. By promoting relaxation and reducing physiological stress markers, earthing may enhance emotional health and wellness and support mental health.

However, while these results are promising, it is important to approach them with caution. Many of the studies on earthing and stress are preliminary and involve small sample sizes. Larger, more rigorous studies are needed to validate these findings and explore how earthing interacts with other factors that influence stress and anxiety.

3. *Effects on Sleep Quality*

Poor sleep quality is a common problem that affects millions of people worldwide. Sleep disturbances are linked to a range of health issues, including impaired cognitive function, weakened immune response, and increased risk of chronic diseases. Earthing has been suggested as a natural method to improve sleep quality by influencing the body's circadian rhythms and promoting relaxation.

Research on earthing and sleep quality began with a pilot study conducted in 2004, which found that participants who used grounding mats while sleeping experienced fewer awakenings during the night and reported feeling more refreshed in the morning. The study also showed a reduction in nighttime cortisol levels, suggesting that earthing helps regulate the body's stress response and supports a healthy sleep-wake cycle.

Subsequent studies have supported these findings, showing that earthing can improve sleep onset, duration, and overall quality. The proposed mechanism is that grounding helps normalise the body's melatonin production by stabilising the autonomic nervous system. Melatonin is a hormone that regulates sleep and is also a powerful antioxidant. Disruptions in melatonin production, such as those caused by EMF exposure, can lead to sleep disturbances and other health issues.

By creating a more stable bioelectrical environment, earthing may help reset the body's internal clock and promote deeper, more restorative sleep. This effect can be particularly beneficial for individuals who suffer from insomnia, jet lag, or irregular sleep patterns.

While existing research on earthing and sleep quality is promising, more studies are needed to fully understand how grounding interacts with other factors that influence sleep, such as light exposure, diet, and physical activity.

Limitations and Areas for Further Research

While research on earthing is promising, it is important to acknowledge its limitations and the need for further study. One of the primary limitations is the small sample size of many existing studies, which makes it difficult to draw definitive conclusions. Larger, randomised controlled trials are needed to confirm the effects of earthing and establish its potential benefits for various health conditions.

Another limitation is the lack of standardised protocols for earthing research. Different studies use varying methods of grounding, such as direct contact with the Earth, the use of grounding mats, or grounding through electrical outlets. This variability makes it challenging to compare results and determine the most effective way to practise earthing.

There is also a need for research on the long-term effects of earthing. Most existing studies focus on short-term outcomes, such as changes in cortisol levels or inflammatory markers after a few hours or days of grounding. Longitudinal studies that track health outcomes over months or years would provide valuable insights into the potential benefits and risks of regular earthing practice.

Additionally, more research is needed to understand the mechanisms behind earthing's effects. While the theory that earthing reduces oxidative stress by providing free electrons is compelling, it is not yet fully understood how these electrons interact with biological systems. Further studies are needed to explore how earthing influences cellular processes, gene expression, and overall bioelectrical function.

Finally, research on specific populations, such as individuals with chronic inflammatory conditions, sleep disorders, or electromagnetic hypersensitivity, would help clarify whether certain groups benefit more from earthing than others. This information would be valuable for healthcare providers in recommending earthing as part of a comprehensive treatment plan.

Overall, while existing research suggests that earthing has potential health benefits, more rigorous studies are needed to validate these findings and provide a clearer understanding of how grounding affects the body.

How Earthing Complements EMF Reduction

Earthing to Counterbalance EMF Effects

Earthing is often recommended as a complementary strategy for reducing the effects of electromagnetic fields (EMF) on the body. While EMF exposure is an inevitable part of modern life, grounding provides a natural way to balance the body's bioelectrical environment and counteract some of the negative effects associated with EMF exposure.

The primary mechanism through which earthing counteracts EMF is by providing the body with free electrons from the Earth's surface. These electrons help neutralise free radicals generated by exposure to EMF, reducing oxidative stress and inflammation. Some researchers suggest that earthing can also stabilise the body's electrical environment, which may be disrupted by constant exposure to artificial electromagnetic fields.

Studies have shown that earthing can reduce physiological markers of stress and inflammation that are often elevated in individuals exposed to high levels of EMF. For example, one study found that grounding during sleep improved autonomic nervous system function and reduced cortisol levels, which are often dysregulated in individuals exposed to chronic EMF.

Additionally, earthing may help improve sleep quality, which can be negatively impacted by EMF exposure. EMF has been shown to disrupt melatonin production and alter sleep patterns, leading to insomnia and reduced sleep quality. Earthing's ability to stabilise the body's electrical environment may help restore natural sleep rhythms and promote more restful sleep.

While earthing cannot block or eliminate EMF exposure, it offers a natural way to mitigate some of the physiological effects associated with EMF. This makes it a valuable addition to other EMF reduction strategies, such as using shielding products, maintaining distance from devices, and turning off Wi-Fi at night.

Synergistic Benefits of Combining Earthing and EMF Reduction

Combining earthing with EMF reduction strategies offers synergistic benefits that can enhance overall health and health and wellness. While EMF reduction focuses on minimising exposure to artificial electromagnetic fields, earthing provides a way to restore the body's natural electrical balance and support physiological function.

One of the key benefits of combining these approaches is the reduction of oxidative stress. EMF exposure is known to increase the production of free radicals, which can lead to oxidative damage and inflammation. Earthing, on the other hand, provides a source of free electrons that neutralise these free radicals, reducing oxidative stress and its associated health risks. By simultaneously reducing EMF exposure and practising earthing, individuals can create a more balanced bioelectrical environment that supports cellular health and function.

Another benefit is the potential improvement in sleep quality. EMF exposure, particularly at night, has been shown to disrupt melatonin production and alter sleep patterns. Turning off Wi-Fi routers and keeping electronic devices away from the bedroom are effective ways to reduce EMF exposure during sleep. Adding earthing to this routine can further enhance sleep quality by promoting relaxation and stabilising the body's circadian rhythms.

For individuals with electromagnetic hypersensitivity (EHS), combining earthing with EMF reduction can provide additional relief. EHS is characterised by a heightened sensitivity to EMF, leading to symptoms such as headaches, fatigue, and cognitive disturbances. While the condition is not fully understood, some research suggests that earthing can help alleviate these symptoms by reducing the body's electrical charge and restoring bioelectrical balance.

In practical terms, combining earthing and EMF reduction can be achieved through a few simple steps. Start by implementing EMF reduction strategies, such as using wired connections instead of Wi-Fi, turning off devices when not in use, and using shielding products in high-EMF areas. Complement these measures with daily earthing practices, such as walking barefoot on natural surfaces or using grounding mats indoors.

By integrating these practices, individuals can create a comprehensive approach to managing EMF exposure and supporting overall health. While more research is needed to fully understand the synergistic benefits of earthing and EMF reduction, existing evidence suggests that these approaches work well together to promote a healthier and more balanced environment.

Practical Ways to practise Earthing

1.   Outdoor Earthing: Walking Barefoot on Grass or Sand

One of the simplest and most effective ways to practise earthingis by walking barefoot on natural surfaces such as grass, sand, or soil. This direct contact with the Earth allows free electrons to flow from the ground into the body, neutralising free radicals and reducing oxidative stress.

To practise outdoor earthing, find a natural, unpolluted area where you can comfortably walk barefoot for at least 15 to 30 minutes. Parks, beaches, and gardens are ideal locations. Ensure that the surface is free of sharp objects and chemicals, such as pesticides or fertilisers, which can negate the benefits of earthing.

Walking barefoot not only facilitates grounding but also provides additional benefits, such as improving balance, strengthening foot muscles, and promoting a sense of relaxation. For those who live in urban areas with limited access to natural surfaces, spending time in parks or nature reserves can provide opportunities for outdoor earthing.

Regular outdoor earthing can be incorporated into your daily routine, such as during morning walks or while gardening. This practice helps maintain a consistent connection to the Earth's energy and supports overall health and health and wellness.

2. Indoor Earthing: Using Grounding Products

For individuals who do not have access to natural outdoor spaces or prefer to practise earthing indoors, grounding products such as mats, sheets, and patches provide a convenient alternative. These products are made from conductive materials that connect to a grounded outlet, allowing free electrons from the Earth to flow into the body.

Grounding mats are commonly used under desks, beds, or seating areas, providing a grounded surface for the body during work, relaxation, or sleep. Grounding sheets are used on beds to create a grounded sleeping environment, which can enhance sleep quality and support overall health.

To use grounding products effectively, ensure that they are connected to a properly grounded outlet or grounding rod. The grounding connection should be tested with a grounding tester to confirm that it is functioning correctly. When using grounding sheets, make sure that they are in direct contact with bare skin, as clothing can reduce conductivity.

Grounding patches, which are small adhesive patches connected to a grounding wire, can be applied to specific areas of the body to target localised pain or inflammation. This can be particularly beneficial for individuals recovering from injuries or dealing with chronic pain conditions.

While indoor grounding products are not a substitute for outdoor earthing, they offer a practical solution for maintaining a grounded connection when outdoor options are not available. Combining indoor and outdoor earthing practices can provide comprehensive benefits and support a balanced bioelectrical environment.

3. Creating a Daily Routine for Earthing

Incorporating earthing into your daily routine can help establish a consistent practice that supports overall health and health and wellness. A typical earthing routine might include a combination of outdoor and indoor grounding practices, depending on your lifestyle and environment.

Start your day with a brief outdoor earthing session, such as walking barefoot on grass or sand for 15 to 30 minutes. This morning practice can help set a positive tone for the day, reduce stress, and promote mental clarity. If you have access to a garden or park, consider making outdoor earthing part of your exercise routine, such as yoga or stretching.

Throughout the day, incorporate indoor grounding practices, especially if you spend long periods sitting at a desk or working on electronic devices. Use a grounding mat under your desk or a grounding pad on your chair to maintain a grounded connection while working. Taking regular breaks to stand on a grounding mat or practice outdoor earthing can also help reduce stress and improve concentration.

In the evening, incorporate earthing into your wind-down routine. Use a grounding sheet or mat while relaxing or sleeping to promote better sleep quality and support recovery from the day's activities. If you experience localised pain or inflammation, consider using grounding patches in targeted areas.

Creating a daily earthing routine does not require drastic lifestyle changes. Simply integrating grounding practices into your existing habits, such as spending time outdoors or using grounding products during work or relaxation, can provide cumulative benefits. Tracking your progress and noting changes in sleep quality, stress levels, and overall health and wellness can help you tailor your routine to meet your specific needs.

By making earthing a regular part of your life, you can establish a connection with the Earth's energy that supports a balanced bioelectrical environment and promotes long-term health.

Clinical Case Study: 50-year-old Man with Chronic Stress and Sleep Issues

Case Introduction and Patient Profile

The patient is a 50-year-old man who has been experiencing chronic stress and sleep disturbances for the past two years. He reports difficulty falling asleep, frequent nighttime awakenings, and waking up feeling unrefreshed. These issues have affected his daily functioning, leading to increased irritability, fatigue, and difficulty concentrating at work.

The patient's lifestyle includes long hours of work in front of a computer, high levels of EMF exposure from electronic devices, and limited time spent outdoors. Concerned about his declining health, the patient sought a holistic approach to improve his sleep quality and reduce stress levels.

Symptoms and Evaluation

The patient reported a history of chronic stress, which he attributed to his demanding work schedule and lack of time for relaxation. He also experienced symptoms of anxiety, such as a racing heart and difficulty unwinding at the end of the day. His sleep problems included trouble falling asleep, frequent awakenings, and feeling tired upon waking.

A comprehensive health evaluation, including a review of his sleep patterns, stress levels, and exposure to environmental factors, revealed that the patient spent most of his day in high-EMF environments. An EMF assessment of his home showed elevated levels of RF and ELF radiation in his bedroom, likely contributing to his sleep disturbances.

Based on these findings, the patient was advised to implement EMF reduction strategies, including turning off electronic devices at night and creating a low-EMF sleeping environment. He was also introduced to earthing as a complementary practice to support stress reduction and improve sleep quality.

Interventions and Outcome

The patient began by implementing EMF reduction strategies, such as turning off his Wi-Fi router at night, using wired connections for his computer, and moving his bed away from electrical outlets. He also started a daily earthing routine, which included a 30-minute barefoot walk in a nearby park every morning and using a grounding mat under his desk during the day.

After two weeks, the patient reported a noticeable improvement in his sleep quality. He found it easier to fall asleep, experienced fewer nighttime awakenings, and felt more rested in the morning. His stress levels also decreased, and he reported feeling calmer and more focused throughout the day.

The patient continued this routine for three months, during which time he noted significant improvements in his overall health and wellness. His anxiety symptoms diminished, and his sleep quality remained consistently good. A follow-up assessment showed lower cortisol levels and improved heart rate variability, indicating better stress management and autonomic function.

This case study illustrates the potential benefits of combining EMF reduction with earthing to address chronic stress and sleep disturbances. By reducing EMF exposure and reestablishing a connection with the Earth's energy, the patient was able to achieve a better state of health and improve his quality of life.

Comprehensive Review and Recommendations

This final section provides a comprehensive review of key concepts covered in this guide, synthesises scientific findings on EMF and earthing, and offers actionable recommendations for managing EMF exposure. It also provides resources and tools to help implement effective strategies and outlines the potential long-term health benefits of reducing EMF exposure and practising earthing. By combining practical steps with ongoing learning and adaptation, individuals can create a healthier, more balanced lifestyle.

Summary: Introduction to Earthing

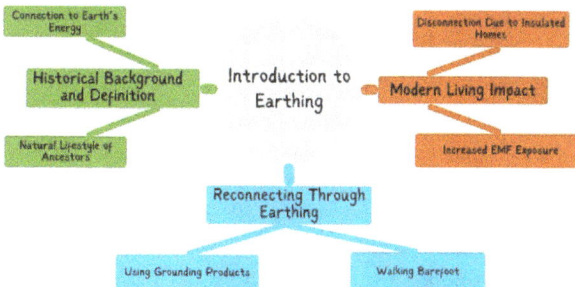

Chapter 7
Recap of Key Concepts

Summary of EMF Health Risks and Misconceptions

Electromagnetic fields (EMF) are ubiquitous in modern life, generated by natural sources like the Earth's magnetic field and human-made sources such as power lines, electronic devices, and wireless communication technologies. Understanding the distinction between different types of EMF—ionising and non-ionising radiation—is critical in assessing their potential health risks.

Ionising radiation (e.g., X-rays and gamma rays) has enough energy to remove tightly bound electrons from atoms, which can lead to cellular and DNA damage. Prolonged exposure to ionising radiation is known to increase the risk of cancer and other serious health conditions. As a result, its use is strictly regulated in medical and industrial settings.

Non-ionising radiation, which includes extremely low-frequency (ELF) fields, radiofrequency (RF) radiation, and microwaves, does not have enough energy to ionise atoms and is generally considered less harmful. However, concerns about the potential health effects of chronic, low-level exposure to non-ionising EMF, particularly from devices like mobile phones, Wi-Fi routers, and smart meters, have led to ongoing research and public debate.

Common misconceptions about EMF include the belief that all EMF exposure is harmful and that products like EMF-blocking beads and pendants can completely eliminate exposure. While certain levels of EMF can pose health risks, most daily exposure falls within safe limits established by international health organisations. Products marketed as EMF shields often lack scientific validation and provide a false sense of security. A more effective approach is to reduce exposure by maintaining distance from devices, limiting usage, and using grounded shielding materials when necessary.

Understanding the nuances of EMF exposure and separating facts from myths is essential for making informed decisions about health and safety.

Key Takeaways from Scientific Research

Scientific research on EMF and its health effects is complex and evolving. While some studies suggest a potential link between prolonged EMF exposure and certain health conditions, such as the increased risk of brain tumours or fertility issues, the evidence is not conclusive. Regulatory agencies like the World Health Organisation (WHO) and the International Commission on Non-Ionising Radiation Protection (ICNIRP) have reviewed existing research and concluded that typical environmental levels of non-ionising radiation are unlikely to cause adverse health effects.

Key findings from scientific research include:

1. **Cancer Risk**: Some epidemiological studies have found a possible association between long-term mobile phone use and certain types of brain tumours, such as gliomas and acoustic neuromas. However, other studies have not found a significant link. The WHO classifies RF radiation as a "possible carcinogen" based on limited evidence, emphasising the need for further research.
2. **Neurological Effects**: Studies on the potential neurological effects of EMF exposure, including impacts on cognitive function and behaviour, have yielded mixed results. Some research suggests that EMF exposure may alter brain activity and sleep patterns, while other studies have not observed significant changes.
3. **Reproductive Health**: Research on EMF exposure and reproductive health has raised concerns about potential effects

on sperm quality and fertility. Some studies indicate that prolonged exposure to RF radiation may reduce sperm motility and viability, but more research is needed to confirm these findings.

4. **Electromagnetic Hypersensitivity (EHS)**: Individuals with EHS report symptoms such as headaches, fatigue, and dizziness in response to EMF exposure. However, double-blind studies have not consistently demonstrated a direct causal relationship between EMF and these symptoms, suggesting that psychological factors may play a role.

Overall, while there is no definitive evidence that typical environmental levels of non-ionising EMF pose serious health risks, ongoing research is necessary to monitor potential long-term effects and explore mechanisms of action.

Practical Strategies for EMF Reduction and Earthing

Reducing EMF exposure and practising earthing can be integrated into daily routines to create a healthier environment. The following practical strategies can help lower exposure and promote overall health and wellness:

1. **Limit EMF Exposure:**
   a. Turn off Wi-Fi routers and other wireless devices when not in use, especially at night.
   b. Use wired connections (e.g., Ethernet cables) for internet access whenever possible.
   c. Keep electronic devices such as mobile phones and tablets at a safe distance from the body, and avoid carrying them in pockets or using them close to the head.
   d. Place large appliances like refrigerators and microwaves away from frequently occupied areas.
2. **Create an EMF-Free Sleeping Environment:**
   a. Remove electronic devices from the bedroom and turn off Wi-Fi routers overnight.

b. Use EMF-shielding materials like bed canopies or shielding paints to reduce RF and ELF radiation in sleeping areas.

3. **Use EMF Shielding Products:**
    a. Shielding products, such as curtains, bed canopies, and grounding mats, can help block or reduce EMF exposure.
    b. Use shielding fabrics and paints to create low-EMF zones in specific areas of the home or workplace.

4. **Practice Earthing:**
    a. Spend at least 15 to 30 minutes each day walking barefoot on natural surfaces like grass, sand, or soil.
    b. Use indoor grounding products, such as mats or sheets, when outdoor earthing is not feasible.

5. **Monitor EMF Levels:**
    a. Use an EMF meter to identify high-EMF areas in the home and implement reduction strategies accordingly.

Integrating these strategies into daily life can create a balanced approach to managing EMF exposure and enhancing overall health.

Developing a Personalised EMF Management Plan

Assessing Your Environment

Developing a personalised EMF management plan begins with assessing your environment to identify sources of EMF and determine areas where exposure can be reduced. An EMF meter can be used to measure radiation levels from various devices, such as Wi-Fi routers, smart meters, and household appliances. Conduct a thorough assessment of your home, starting with bedrooms, living areas, and workspaces, to identify high-EMF areas.

During the assessment, consider the following factors:

1. **Proximity to EMF Sources**: Determine how close frequently used areas are to high-EMF sources like routers, power lines, or large appliances.

2. **Duration of Exposure**: Note how much time is spent near EMF sources, such as working in front of a computer or using a mobile phone.
3. **Environmental Factors**: Consider structural elements like electrical wiring and the presence of nearby cell towers, which can contribute to ambient EMF levels.

Document your findings and highlight areas where EMF exposure is highest. This information will guide the implementation of reduction strategies and help prioritise changes.

Implementing Strategies Based on Individual Needs

Once you have assessed your environment, develop a customised plan to reduce EMF exposure based on your individual needs and lifestyle. Focus on areas with the highest levels of EMF and the most prolonged exposure.

1. **For the Home:**
   a. Create low-EMF zones in frequently used spaces, such as bedrooms and living rooms, by using shielding products and turning off devices when not in use.
   b. Rearrange furniture to maintain a safe distance from high-EMF sources, such as microwaves and televisions.
2. **For the Workplace:**
   a. Position your workstation away from high-EMF sources like electrical panels or routers.
   b. Use wired connections instead of Wi-Fi for internet access.
3. **For Personal Devices:**
   a. Use EMF-blocking phone and laptop cases and keep devices in aeroplane mode when not in use.
   b. Limit the use of Bluetooth and wireless peripherals, and switch to wired options when possible.
4. **For Sensitive Individuals:**
   a. Individuals with electromagnetic hypersensitivity (EHS) may benefit from more stringent measures, such as

creating a completely shielded sleeping area and using grounding products regularly.

Tailor your plan to suit your unique circumstances and involve family members to ensure that everyone benefits from a reduced EMF environment.

Monitoring and Adjusting Over Time

An effective EMF management plan requires regular monitoring and adjustment to ensure continued effectiveness. Use an EMF meter to periodically reassess radiation levels in your home and workplace, especially after making changes such as moving furniture, adding new devices, or implementing shielding products.

Monitor your health and health and wellness, noting any changes in symptoms, sleep quality, or overall energy levels. Adjust your plan based on these observations:

1. **If EMF Levels Increase:**
   a. Investigate potential new sources of EMF, such as recently installed appliances or nearby cell tower upgrades.
   b. Implement additional shielding or reduce device usage in affected areas.
2. **If Health Symptoms Persist:**
   a. Consider consulting with a healthcare professional or EMF specialist for further guidance.
   b. Explore additional earthing practices or alternative methods to enhance health and health and wellness.

Over time, make adjustments to your plan to reflect changes in your environment, lifestyle, or health status. Keeping a log of EMF measurements and health observations can help track progress and identify trends, allowing you to refine your approach.

Resources and Tools for Managing EMF Exposure

Recommended Products and Tools for EMF Reduction

Several products and tools can help manage EMF exposure effectively:

1. **EMF Meters**: Use an EMF meter to identify high-EMF areas and measure the effectiveness of reduction strategies. Recommended brands include Trifield and Cornet.
2. **Shielding Products**: Shielding paints (e.g., YSHIELD), fabrics, bed canopies, and curtains are effective for blocking RF and ELF radiation. Use these products in high-EMF areas like bedrooms and home offices.
3. **Grounding Products**: Grounding mats, sheets, and patches can help restore the body's natural electrical balance. Recommended products include those from brands like Earthing and Grounded Wellbeing.
4. **EMF-Blocking Phone and Laptop Cases**: Cases made with conductive materials can reduce direct RF exposure. Brands like Defender Shield offer a range of options.

Using these products, along with lifestyle changes, can significantly reduce EMF exposure and create a healthier living environment.

Books, Reports, and Research Papers for Further Reading

For individuals interested in learning more about EMF and earthing, the following resources are recommended:

1. **Books:**
   a. *EMF* by Dr. Joseph Mercola – A comprehensive guide to understanding and mitigating EMF exposure.
   b. *Earthing: The Most Important Health Discovery Ever?* by Clinton Ober, Stephen T. Sinatra, and Martin Zucker – An in-depth exploration of the benefits of grounding.

2. **Reports:**
   a. *BioInitiative Report 2012* – A scientific review of EMF and its health effects.
   b. *World Health Organisation (WHO) Fact Sheets on EMF* – Provides an overview of EMF exposure guidelines and health risks.

3. **Research Papers:**
   a. Research studies published in journals like *Journal of Environmental and Public Health* and *Bioelectromagnetics* offer insights into the health effects of EMF and the benefits of earthing.

These resources provide a solid foundation for understanding the science behind EMF and earthing and offer practical advice for managing exposure.

Long-Term Health Benefits of EMF Reduction and Earthing

Improved Sleep, Reduced Stress, and Better Overall Health

Reducing EMF exposure and practising earthing can lead to a range of long-term health benefits, including improved sleep quality, reduced stress levels, and better overall health. By creating a low-EMF environment and reconnecting with the Earth's natural energy, individuals can support their body's natural rhythms and enhance physical and mental health and wellness.

1. **Improved Sleep**: Lowering EMF exposure, especially at night, can help regulate melatonin production and support a healthy sleep-wake cycle. Practising earthing has been shown to reduce nighttime cortisol levels, leading to deeper, more restorative sleep.

2. **Reduced Stress**: Earthing can stabilise the autonomic nervous system, reducing physiological markers of stress such as elevated heart rate and cortisol levels. Combined with EMF reduction, this can lead to better stress management and emotional resilience.

3. **Better Overall Health**: Lowering oxidative stress and inflammation through earthing and minimising EMF exposure can reduce the risk of chronic diseases, improve immune function, and enhance overall vitality.

By integrating these practices into daily life, individuals can experience lasting health benefits and improve their quality of life.

Creating a Balanced and Grounded Lifestyle

Creating a balanced and grounded lifestyle involves making conscious choices to reduce EMF exposure and incorporate earthing into daily routines. It is about finding a balance between enjoying the conveniences of modern technology and maintaining a connection to the Earth's natural energy.

Simple practices like turning off devices when not in use, using wired connections, spending time outdoors, and using grounding products can make a significant difference in overall health and wellness. Educating family members and creating a collective effort to reduce EMF exposure can lead to a healthier home environment and support long-term health.

A balanced and grounded lifestyle fosters a sense of harmony between the technological and natural worlds, promoting a state of health and wellness that aligns with the body's natural rhythms.

Final Thoughts and Future Directions

The Evolving Field of EMF Research

The field of EMF research is continually evolving as new technologies emerge and our understanding of EMF exposure grows. Researchers are exploring various aspects of EMF, from its potential health effects to effective mitigation strategies. As technology advances, it is crucial to remain informed and adapt our approaches to managing EMF exposure.

Ongoing research is focusing on the long-term effects of chronic low-level EMF exposure, particularly in vulnerable populations such as children and individuals with pre-existing health conditions. Studies are also examining the cumulative impact of simultaneous exposure to multiple EMF sources, such as mobile phones, Wi-Fi routers, and smart meters.

New findings will continue to shape public health guidelines and recommendations for safe EMF exposure levels. It is important to stay up-to-date with emerging research and consider incorporating new strategies and products as they become available.

Encouraging Ongoing Learning and Adaptation

As our understanding of EMF and its effects evolves, so too should our approach to managing exposure. Ongoing learning and adaptation are essential for maintaining a healthy balance in an increasingly technology-driven world.

Stay informed by regularly reviewing credible sources, attending webinars or workshops, and consulting with experts in the field. Encourage open discussions with family members, healthcare providers, and community leaders about EMF management and earthing practices.

Embracing a proactive and informed approach will help individuals make better decisions about their health and health and wellness in the context of modern technology.

Glossary

1. **Electromagnetic Fields (EMF)**

    An area of energy that is produced by electrically charged
    objects. EMF can be classified into ionising and non-ionising
    radiation, depending on its frequency and energy levels.
    Sources of EMF include natural phenomena like the Earth's
    magnetic field and human-made sources such as electronic
    devices, power lines, and wireless communication
    technologies.

2. **Ionising Radiation**

    A type of electromagnetic radiation with high energy levels
    that can remove tightly bound electrons from atoms, causing
    ionisation. Examples include X-rays, gamma rays, and some
    ultraviolet (UV) rays. Prolonged exposure to ionising radiation
    can cause cellular and DNA damage, increasing the risk of
    cancer and other health issues.

3. **Non-Ionising Radiation**

    A type of electromagnetic radiation with lower energy levels
    that does not have enough energy to ionise atoms or
    molecules. Examples include radiofrequency (RF) radiation
    from mobile phones and Wi-Fi routers, as well as extremely
    low-frequency (ELF) fields from power lines and household
    appliances.

4. **Radiofrequency (RF) Radiation**

    A form of non-ionising radiation emitted by wireless
    communication devices such as mobile phones, Wi-Fi routers,
    and Bluetooth devices. RF radiation is used to transmit data
    over short and long distances.

5. Extremely Low-Frequency (ELF) Radiation

A form of non-ionising radiation emitted by power lines, electrical wiring, and household appliances. ELF radiation has very low frequencies, typically below 300 Hz, and is commonly found in the home and workplace.

6. Electromagnetic Hypersensitivity (EHS)

A condition in which individuals report a range of symptoms, such as headaches, fatigue, and dizziness, that they believe are caused by exposure to electromagnetic fields. While the symptoms are real, scientific studies have not consistently demonstrated a direct causal relationship between EMF exposure and these symptoms.

7. Grounding (Earthing)

A practice that involves direct physical contact with the Earth's surface, such as walking barefoot on grass or using grounding products indoors. Grounding is believed to allow electrons to flow from the Earth into the body, neutralising free radicals and reducing oxidative stress, inflammation, and overall stress.

8. Shielding

The use of materials that block or reflect electromagnetic radiation to reduce exposure. Shielding products include bed canopies, curtains, fabrics, paints, and window films made from conductive materials like silver or copper.

9. Free Radicals

Highly reactive molecules with unpaired electrons that can cause oxidative stress and damage to cells. Free radicals are naturally produced in the body during normal metabolic processes and in response to environmental factors such as

EMF exposure. Antioxidants and grounding practices can help neutralise free radicals.

10. Oxidative Stress

A state of imbalance between free radicals and antioxidants in the body, leading to cellular damage. Chronic oxidative stress is linked to various health problems, including inflammation, cardiovascular disease, and neurodegenerative disorders.

11. Melatonin

A hormone produced by the pineal gland in response to darkness. Melatonin regulates the sleep-wake cycle and has antioxidant properties. EMF exposure has been shown to disrupt melatonin production, leading to sleep disturbances.

12. Heart Rate Variability (HRV)

A measure of the variation in time between consecutive heartbeats, reflecting the body's ability to adapt to stress and changes in the environment. Higher HRV is associated with better health and resilience to stress, while lower HRV is linked to chronic stress and poor health outcomes.

13. Faraday Cage

An enclosure made from conductive materials, such as metal mesh, that blocks electromagnetic fields by creating a protective barrier. Bed canopies made from conductive fabrics function as Faraday cages to shield against radiofrequency radiation.

14. Bioelectrical Environment

The body's internal electrical environment, is influenced by the flow of ions and electrical charges within cells and tissues. The bioelectrical environment plays a role in various physiological processes, including nerve conduction, muscle contraction, and cellular signalling.

15. Cortisol

A hormone produced by the adrenal glands in response to stress. Cortisol levels follow a diurnal rhythm, peaking in the morning and gradually decreasing throughout the day. Dysregulated cortisol rhythms are associated with chronic stress, sleep disturbances, and anxiety.

16. Circadian Rhythms

The body's internal clock regulates the sleep-wake cycle, hormone production, and other physiological processes based on a 24-hour cycle. Disruptions to circadian rhythms, such as those caused by EMF exposure or irregular sleep patterns, can affect overall health and health and wellness.

17. Free Electrons

Negatively charged particles that are present on the surface of the Earth. Grounding practices allow these free electrons to flow into the body, potentially reducing oxidative stress and supporting the body's natural electrical balance.

18. Conductivity

The ability of a material to allow the flow of electrical current. Conductive materials, such as metals and certain fabrics, are used in shielding products to block or redirect electromagnetic radiation.

19. Diurnal Rhythm

The natural pattern of physiological processes, such as hormone production and body temperature, that follow a 24-hour cycle based on light and darkness. Cortisol and melatonin are two hormones that exhibit diurnal rhythms.

20. BioInitiative Report

A comprehensive review of scientific research on EMF and its health effects, was first published in 2007 and updated in 2012. The report summarises studies on the biological effects of EMF and provides recommendations for exposure limits.

References

A. Electromagnetic Fields (EMF)

An area of energy produced by electrically charged objects. EMF can be classified into ionising and non-ionising radiation, depending on its frequency and energy levels. Sources of EMF include natural phenomena like the Earth's magnetic field and human-made sources such as electronic devices, power lines, and wireless communication technologies.

References:

1. World Health Organisation (WHO). "Electromagnetic Fields and Public Health."
2. National Institute of Environmental Health Sciences (NIEHS). "Electric and Magnetic Fields."
3. BioInitiative Report. "A Rationale for Biologically-Based Public Exposure Standards for Electromagnetic Fields (ELF and RF)."

B. Ionising Radiation

A type of electromagnetic radiation with high energy levels that can remove tightly bound electrons from atoms, causing ionisation. Examples include X-rays, gamma rays, and some ultraviolet (UV) rays. Prolonged exposure to ionising radiation can cause cellular and DNA damage, increasing the risk of cancer and other health issues.

References:

4. International Commission on Radiological Protection (ICRP). "Protection Against Ionising Radiation."

5. National Cancer Institute. "Radiation and Cancer."

6. United States Environmental Protection Agency (EPA). "Ionising Radiation and Health Effects."

C. Non-Ionising Radiation

A type of electromagnetic radiation with lower energy levels that does not have enough energy to ionise atoms or molecules. Examples include radiofrequency (RF) radiation from mobile phones and Wi-Fi routers, as well as extremely low-frequency (ELF) fields from power lines and household appliances.

References:

7. World Health Organisation (WHO). "Non-Ionising Radiation, Part 2: Radiofrequency Electromagnetic Fields."

8. International Agency for Research on Cancer (IARC). "IARC Monographs on the Evaluation of Carcinogenic Risks to Humans: Non-Ionising Radiation."

9. National Institute for Occupational Safety and Health (NIOSH). "EMF: Electric and Magnetic Fields Associated with the Use of Electric Power."

D. Radiofrequency (RF) Radiation

A form of non-ionising radiation emitted by wireless communication devices such as mobile phones, Wi-Fi routers, and Bluetooth devices. RF radiation is used to transmit data over short and long distances.

References:

10. Federal Communications Commission (FCC). "Radio Frequency Safety."

11. Health Protection Agency (HPA). "Health Effects from Radiofrequency Electromagnetic Fields."

12. National Toxicology Programme (NTP). "Report on Carcinogens: RF Radiation."

E. Extremely Low-Frequency (ELF) Radiation

A form of non-ionising radiation emitted by power lines, electrical wiring, and household appliances. ELF radiation has very low frequencies, typically below 300 Hz, and is commonly found in the home and workplace.

References:

13. World Health Organisation (WHO). "Extremely Low Frequency Fields."

14. European Commission. "Exposure to Electromagnetic Fields (EMF): The Role of the European Union."

15. International Agency for Research on Cancer (IARC). "Monographs on the Evaluation of Carcinogenic Risks to Humans: ELF Electric and Magnetic Fields."

F. Electromagnetic Hypersensitivity (EHS)

A condition in which individuals report a range of symptoms, such as headaches, fatigue, and dizziness, that they believe are caused by exposure to electromagnetic fields. While the symptoms are real, scientific studies have not consistently demonstrated a direct causal relationship between EMF exposure and these symptoms.

References:

16. Rubin, G. J., et al. "Electromagnetic Hypersensitivity: A Systematic Review of Provocation Studies." *Psychosomatic Medicine*.

17. Leitgeb, N., and Schröttner, J. "Electromagnetic Hypersensitivity (EHS) and Subjective Health Complaints

Associated with Electromagnetic Fields of Mobile Communications." *Bioelectromagnetics.*

18. Dieudonné, M. "Does Electromagnetic Hypersensitivity Originate from Nocebo Responses? Indications from a Qualitative Study." *Bioelectromagnetics.*

G. Grounding (Earthing)

A practice that involves direct physical contact with the Earth's surface, such as walking barefoot on grass or using grounding products indoors. Grounding is believed to allow electrons to flow from the Earth into the body, neutralising free radicals and reducing oxidative stress, inflammation, and overall stress.

References:

19. Ober, C., Sinatra, S., and Zucker, M. "Earthing: The Most Important Health Discovery Ever?"

20. Chevalier, G., et al. "The Effect of Earthing (Grounding) on Human Physiology." *Journal of Environmental and Public Health.*

21. Sokal, K., and Sokal, P. "Earthing the Human Body Influences Physiologic Processes." *Journal of Alternative and Complementary Medicine.*

H. Shielding

The use of materials that block or reflect electromagnetic radiation to reduce exposure. Shielding products include bed canopies, curtains, fabrics, paints, and window films made from conductive materials like silver or copper.

References:

22. YSHIELD EMR Protection. "EMF Shielding Products for Home and Office."

23. Shielding Solutions Ltd. "EMF Shielding Paints and Fabrics."

24. Panagopoulos, D. J., and Margaritis, L. H. "The Effect of Shielding on the Biological Impact of Electromagnetic Fields." *Electromagnetic Biology and Medicine.*

I. Free Radicals

Highly reactive molecules with unpaired electrons that can cause oxidative stress and damage to cells. Free radicals are naturally produced in the body during normal metabolic processes and in response to environmental factors such as EMF exposure. Antioxidants and grounding practices can help neutralise free radicals.

References:

25. Halliwell, B. "Free Radicals and Antioxidants: Updating a Personal View." *Nutrition Reviews.*

26. Lobo, V., et al. "Free Radicals, Antioxidants, and Functional Foods: Impact on Human Health." *Pharmacognosy Reviews.*

27. Valko, M., et al. "Free Radicals and Antioxidants in Normal Physiological Functions and Human Disease." *International Journal of Biochemistry & Cell Biology.*

J. Oxidative Stress

A state of imbalance between free radicals and antioxidants in the body, leading to cellular damage. Chronic oxidative stress is linked to various health problems, including inflammation, cardiovascular disease, and neurodegenerative disorders.

References:

28. Finkel, T., and Holbrook, N. J. "Oxidants, Oxidative Stress, and the Biology of Ageing." *Nature.*

29. Birben, E., et al. "Oxidative Stress and Antioxidant Defense." *World Allergy Organisation Journal.*

30. Uttara, B., et al. "Oxidative Stress and Neurodegenerative Diseases: A Review of Upstream and Downstream Antioxidant Therapeutic Options." *Current Neuropharmacology.*

K. Melatonin

A hormone produced by the pineal gland in response to darkness. Melatonin regulates the sleep-wake cycle and has antioxidant properties. EMF exposure has been shown to disrupt melatonin production, leading to sleep disturbances.

References:

31. Arendt, J. "Melatonin, Circadian Rhythms, and Sleep." *New England Journal of Medicine.*

32. Reiter, R. J. "Melatonin: Clinical Relevance." *Best Practice & Research Clinical Endocrinology & Metabolism.*

33. Halgamuge, M. N. "Pineal Melatonin Level Disruption in Humans Due to Electromagnetic Fields and Ions." *Bioelectromagnetics.*

L. Heart Rate Variability (HRV)

A measure of the variation in time between consecutive heartbeats, reflecting the body's ability to adapt to stress and changes in the environment. Higher HRV is associated with better health and resilience to stress, while lower HRV is linked to chronic stress and poor health outcomes.

References:

34. Shaffer, F., and Ginsberg, J. P. "An Overview of Heart Rate Variability Metrics and Norms." *Frontiers in Public Health.*

35. Thayer, J. F., et al. "The Effects of Heart Rate Variability on Health and Health and wellness: A Systematic Review of Biological, Psychological, and Social Processes." *Neuroscience & Biobehavioural Reviews.*

36. McCraty, R., and Shaffer, F. "Heart Rate Variability: New Perspectives on Physiological Mechanisms, Assessment of Self-Regulatory Capacity, and Health Risk." *Global Advances in Health and Medicine.*

M. Faraday Cage

An enclosure made from conductive materials, such as metal mesh, that blocks electromagnetic fields by creating a protective barrier. Bed canopies made from conductive fabrics function as Faraday cages to shield against radiofrequency radiation.

References:

37. Christensen, C. "Faraday Cages: Theory and Application." *IEEE Antennas and Propagation Magazine.*

38. Marcus, G. "Faraday Cages and Their Use in Modern Technology." *Physics Review Letters.*

39. Wood, R. "Practical Use of Faraday Cages in Biomedical Research." *Journal of Biomedical Engineering.*

N. Bioelectrical Environment

The body's internal electrical environment, is influenced by the flow of ions and electrical charges within cells and tissues. The bioelectrical environment plays a role in various physiological processes, including nerve conduction, muscle contraction, and cellular signalling.

References:

40. Becker, R. O., and Selden, G. "The Body Electric: Electromagnetism and the Foundation of Life."

41. Szent-Györgyi, A. "Bioelectronics and the Bioelectrical Environment." *Journal of Bioenergetics and Biomembranes.*

42. Pilla, A. A. "Mechanisms and Therapeutic Applications of Time-Varying and Static Magnetic Fields." *Electromagnetic Biology and Medicine.*

O. Cortisol

A hormone produced by the adrenal glands in response to stress. Cortisol levels follow a diurnal rhythm, peaking in the morning and gradually decreasing throughout the day. Dysregulated cortisol rhythms are associated with chronic stress, sleep disturbances, and anxiety.

References:

43. Sapolsky, R. M., Romero, L. M., and Munck, A. U. "How Do Glucocorticoids Influence Stress Responses? Integrating Permissive, Suppressive, Stimulatory, and Preparative Actions." *Endocrine Reviews.*

44. McEwen, B. S. "Stress, Adaptation, and Disease: Allostasis and Allostatic Load." *Annals of the New York Academy of Sciences.*

45. Chrousos, G. P., and Gold, P. W. "The Concepts of Stress and Stress System Disorders: Overview of Physical and Behavioural Homeostasis." *JAMA.*

P. Circadian Rhythms

The body's internal clock regulates the sleep-wake cycle, hormone production, and other physiological processes based on a 24-hour cycle. Disruptions to circadian rhythms, such as those caused by EMF exposure or irregular sleep patterns, can affect overall health and health and wellness.

References:

46. Czeisler, C. A., and Gooley, J. J. "Sleep and Circadian Rhythms in Humans." *Cold Spring Harbor Symposia on Quantitative Biology*.

47. Foster, R. G., and Kreitzman, L. "Circadian Rhythms: A Very Short Introduction."

48. Bass, J., and Takahashi, J. S. "Circadian Integration of Metabolism and Energetics." *Science*.

Q. Free Electrons

Negatively charged particles that are present on the surface of the Earth. Grounding practices allow these free electrons to flow into the body, potentially reducing oxidative stress and supporting the body's natural electrical balance.

References:

49. Chevalier, G., and Sinatra, S. T. "Grounding the Human Body Reduces Blood Viscosity—a Major Factor in Cardiovascular Disease." *Journal of Alternative and Complementary Medicine*.

50. Ober, C., Sinatra, S. T., and Zucker, M. "Earthing: Health Implications of Reconnecting the Human Body to the Earth's Surface Electrons." *Journal of Environmental and Public Health*.

51. Ghaly, M., and Teplitz, D. "The Biologic Effects of Grounding the Human Body During Sleep as Measured by Cortisol Levels and Subjective Reporting of Sleep, Pain, and Stress." *Journal of Alternative and Complementary Medicine*.

R. Conductivity

The ability of a material to allow the flow of electrical current. Conductive materials, such as metals and certain fabrics, are used in shielding products to block or redirect electromagnetic radiation.

References:

52. Gabriel, C., and Gabriel, S. "Dielectric Properties of Biological Tissue: Variation with Age." *Physics in Medicine and Biology*.

53. Schwan, H. P. "Electrical Properties of Tissues and Cell Suspensions: Mechanisms and Models." *Annual Review of Biophysics and Bioengineering*.

54. Martinsen, Ø. G., Grimnes, S., and Schwan, H. P. "Interface Phenomena and Dielectric Properties of Biological Tissues." *Encyclopedia of Surface and Colloid Science*.

S. Diurnal Rhythm

The natural pattern of physiological processes, such as hormone production and body temperature, that follow a 24-hour cycle based on light and darkness. Cortisol and melatonin are two hormones that exhibit diurnal rhythms.

References:

55. Scheer, F. A., Hilton, M. F., Mantzoros, C. S., and Shea, S. A. "Adverse Metabolic and Cardiovascular Consequences of Circadian Misalignment." *Proceedings of the National Academy of Sciences*.

56. Buxton, O. M., and Marcelli, E. "Short and Long Sleep Are Positively Associated with Obesity, Diabetes, Hypertension, and Cardiovascular Disease in Adults." *Social Science & Medicine.*

57. Cajochen, C. "Effects of Light on Human Circadian Rhythms, Sleep, and Mood." *Seminars in Perinatology.*

T. BioInitiative Report

A comprehensive review of scientific research on EMF and its health effects, was first published in 2007 and updated in 2012. The report summarises studies on the biological effects of EMF and provides recommendations for exposure limits.

References:

58. BioInitiative Report 2012. "A Rationale for Biologically-Based Public Exposure Standards for Electromagnetic Fields (ELF and RF)."

59. Carpenter, D. O., and Sage, C. "Setting Prudent Public Health Policy for Electromagnetic Field Exposures." *Reviews on Environmental Health.*

60. Sage, C., and Burgio, E. "Electromagnetic Fields, Pulsed Radiofrequency Radiation, and Epigenetics: How Wireless Technologies May Affect Childhood Development." *Child Development.*

www.ingramcontent.com/pod-product-compliance
Lightning Source LLC
Chambersburg PA
CBHW071242020426

42333CB00015B/1590